EAT FREELY

GOD'S PERSPECTIVE ABOUT FOOD

KAREN BROOKS

CONTENTS

Paperback: 978-1-951694-14-2
Ebook: 978-1-951694-16-6

For permissions, bulk order requests and price schedule contact:
admin@gracepointpublishing.com
GracePoint books may be purchased for educational, business, or sales promotional use. This book is not intended as a substitute for the medical advice of a physician or qualified therapist. The reader should regularly consult a physician in matters relating to his/her health and particularly with respect to any symptoms that may require diagnosis or medical attention.

Artwork by Madi Edgar Photography by Jennifer A. Steiger Edited by Spiral Up Designs, Susie Biggs Colorado Springs, CO
Published by GracePoint Matrix, LLC publishing Division
GracePointpublishing.com GraceLight Press 322 N. Tejon St.
Colorado Springs, CO 80903

DEDICATION

This book is dedicated to anyone who has ever struggled, in any way, with food. I pray you find your freedom (Luke 4:18).

ACKNOWLEDGMENTS

To my husband and best friend, Chris Brooks, this book undoubtedly would not have been possible without you. Your unwavering love and support help me realize goals and dreams that seem beyond my reach. You believe in me even when I don't. You continually encourage me to be exactly who God created me to be. Thank you for never letting go of my hand. Love you. It's 10:14.

To my parents, Ronald and Patricia Peterson, thank you for a lifetime of undeniable love and sacrifice. You've provided me with a strong foundation giving me latitude to see things from different perspectives and permission to ask lots of questions. The childhood you gave me is a priceless gift that I will never be able to repay. I love you both more than words can say.

To my mother-in-law, Sandy Brooks, thank you for always being my reference and for your willingness to share your

Biblical expertise and insight whenever I have one of my questions. It always leads to deep conversations that I truly cherish. I love you.

To my editor, Michelle Vandepas, thank you for patiently walking me through this book-writing process. I believe our meeting was a divine connection!

To GracePoint Publishing, thank you for believing in me and in this book.

To my dear friends, Anne Evans and Judy Ringgold, thank you for making the time to read, edit and provide comment on the final manuscript (even though you had to number the pages). Your fresh perspectives were unique and exactly what I was looking for.

To my cover designer and adopted family member, "Madi Moon" Edgar, thank you for being able to turn my thoughts into your beautiful designs. You have a creative talent that I am grateful you're willing to share.

To my North Carolina neighbors and dear friends, Jack and Sara Carroll, thank you for always being available when I needed "an opinion."

PREFACE

For several years I have known I was going to write this book. During that time, the Lord had been routinely bringing food-related topics to my mind. Before this, I never had a desire to write a book. I never even considered it. In my lifetime, I have written quite frequently. But nothing of the level of a book. Most of my writing consisted of the often-passed notes to friends during middle school and high school, class-assigned essays, reports, and, most recently, a master's thesis. One research paper I wrote during college regarding eating disorders was recommended for publishing by my sociology professor, but I never pursued it. While living out the 9-to-5 of corporate America, I wrote a fair number of contracts and legal documents. But never once did I imagine writing a book.

Initially, I decided to write this book for an audience of one: myself. I was tired of being confused about food. The constant questioning of what to eat, when to eat, and how much to eat consumed my thoughts. Navigating those questions became a bit of an obsession. Food rules began dictating my life. I fell into an unhealthy cycle of researching, implementing, revamping, and trial and error, followed by failing to get the results I wanted. The worst part was finding out the advice I was following was incorrect or had been changed recently.

Simply put, I had had enough. As a Christian, I learned that the Bible was the source of spiritual guidance. I knew it was the guidebook to get into heaven, yet I began noticing the Bible addressed the topic of food. Food is mentioned all through the Bible. In all my studying and researching, I never considered the Bible as a nutritional reference source. Naturally, I wanted to find out if the Good Book could also serve as a physical guide to eating.

Piggybacking off my lifelong exposure to the church and my passion for nutrition and health, I began researching the Bible for food references. After graduating with my master's degree in August 2018, my husband and I took a vacation to Florida. Since I was no longer studying, I planned to read the Bible from cover to cover or from Genesis to Revelation. Reading the Bible from beginning to end in a year is a typical resolution many Christians would attempt. Some can even tell you a how many times they have accomplished this exercise. Parenthetically, as I write this book, I've yet to achieve that one. Anyway, while reading the Bible from beginning to end, I planned to pay attention to all food references I encountered. But oddly, I spent a significant amount of time in Genesis studying Adam and Eve in the Garden of Eden. I also spent a considerable amount of time in the Gospels of the New Testament studying the Crucifixion.

Realizing I was falling far behind on my "read the entire Bible" goal, I commented to my husband on several occasions that I could not seem to get out of the Garden or away from the cross. My husband simply said, "Well, maybe that's where the Lord wants you to focus." Surrendering what I thought was the right way to research the topic and instead following the Lord's leading, He showed me that the Garden of Eden and, ultimately, the Crucifixion is pivotal in determining a Christian's relationship to the food we eat.

I earned my Master's in Nutrition and Human Performance, hoping to understand food better and how we were to consume it. I quickly determined that the science of nutrition is incredibly complex. But then I wondered why should a person who is responsible for feeding himself or herself every day need an advanced degree to do it correctly? Finding the answer to this question seemed even more critical, considering that the consequences of doing it wrong can be extraordinarily costly.

Presently, I am an entrepreneur. I own a business helping clients with the impact of structural, emotional, and nutritional stress. Most of the people who come into my office complain that food makes them feel bad or they just do not know what to eat. I get it. The relationship with food has become incredibly dysfunctional. Over time, it seems that every person reaches the point where they simply get tired of trying or at least tired of trying to figure it out.

There is a quote believed to be made by Hippocrates,

commonly referred to as the Father of Medicine, and often attributed to the Bible that says, "Let your food be your medicine." Hippocrates, who was born around 460 BC, believed that medicine should be separate and apart from religion. Sickness was not a punishment from an angry god. Instead, it was the result of several external factors, including the environment. Because of that belief, I submit that this could be the origin of a misguided way of thinking. If food is your medicine and medicine should be separate from religion, then food should be separate from religion as well. It seems that this is still the prevailing belief in our culture today. But according to the Bible, food is intricately connected to religion or at least to Jesus. Food is vitally important. We need it for health. We need it to survive. But how do we get back to a healthy relationship with food? Or better yet, how did the relationship become dysfunctional?

To begin, it is important to know what food is. According to the Federal Food, Drug and Cosmetic Act of 21 U. S. Code § 321 section entitled "Definitions; generally", food is defined as "(1) articles used for food or drink for man or other animals, (2) chewing gum, and (3) articles used for components of any such article." I don't know about you, but I didn't find that definition particularly helpful. So, I looked for other definitions. According to Merriam-Webster, food is a "material consisting essentially of protein, carbohydrate, and fat used in the body of an organism to sustain growth, repair, and vital processes and to furnish energy." The definition provides even more detail to include "such food together with supplementary substances (such as minerals, vitamins, and condiments)." Admittedly, from a nutritionist perspective, this definition seems complete. A quick Google search for "food definition" will provide you with several responses of varying detail. Suffice it to say that there is no real consensus.

How does the Bible define food? In Genesis 1:29 God tells Adam, "I give you every seed-bearing plant on the face of the whole earth and every tree that has fruit with seed in it. They will be yours for food." Adam could eat any fruit in the Garden except that of the Tree of the Knowledge of Good and Evil. God goes even further by stating that "And to all the beasts of the earth and all the birds in the sky and all the creatures that move along the ground—everything that has the breath of life in it—I give every green plant for food." God provided food for everything He created. What I found interesting was what God did not say. He didn't tell Adam about the protein, carbohydrate, and fat content of each fruit. He didn't go into detail of the vitamin, mineral, and enzyme content. Maybe because Adam didn't need to know. The food was for Adam to enjoy. Think about that for a moment. Taking this a step further, God gave Adam the responsibility of naming all the animals. In Genesis 2:19, we read, "He brought them to the man to see what he would name them; and whatever the man called each living creature, that was its name." Adam was smart enough to remember them all. Yet, God did not see the need for Adam to know the nutritional content of each food item in the Garden.

Then after the Flood, in Genesis 9:3, God tells Noah, going forward, "Everything that lives and moves about will be food for you. Just as I gave you the green plants, I now give you everything." However, just like in the Garden when God told Adam to eat freely, except... He tells Noah, I give you everything, but ... There was a requirement when the meat was eaten; it was to be cooked.

There is a beautiful simplicity in the Biblical definition of food. It is a simplicity I believe we are craving today. It's not about how much protein or fat the food contains. Rather, simply eat seed-bearing plants and fruit and eat meat from animals that have eaten green plants. I hope that after reading this book, you, too, will recognize God's original plan for man's relationship with food and the corresponding relationship with Him. While food is necessary for our survival, too much emphasis has been placed on its connection with our health, thus taking away emphasis from the Gift-giver Himself. When Adam and Eve sinned, it changed our spiritual condition. Jesus came and paid that debt. But arguably, the sin changed our relationship to food as well. Jesus's death on the cross fixed it.

This book has been consuming my thoughts for the last several years. I believe that the Lord has been showing me glimpses of His nutritional plan. He created food. He spoke it into existence. Lovingly, He used food to bring us back to a right relationship with Him. He doesn't want us to stress over what to eat. He tells us not to worry about it. But through gifts that we received because of the cross, such as grace, righteousness, faith, peace, wisdom, thanksgiving, seeds, and communion, our physical relationship with food and health changed as well.

The Bible is not just a book that teaches spiritual living.

Nor does it only take effect the moment you die. It is a guidebook drawing us into a more profound and sweeter relationship with our Heavenly Father, who designed us to need food daily.

There is a misconception that science and the Bible are opposed. In some instances, maybe so. But regarding food, science is beginning to prove what the Bible has always said: Eat what God created. Just because something is edible does not mean it can be considered food. We are not designed to function on ingestible items produced in a lab. According to vocabulary.com, food is "anything that you can eat and digest." The word "anything" leaves the definition of food open to interpretation. Part of the struggle we have with eating is that we don't know what constitutes food.

This book is not a guidebook on what to eat. There are more books about that in bookstores than can be counted. Add to the books the vast number of sites to be researched on the Internet. Understandably, people want to know what to eat. Truthfully, they need to know. I believe that the perspective is wrong. It's not about a magic combination of macronutrients or the accompanying vitamins and minerals. It's the relationship to the Food Creator. This book is more of a guidebook on how to see food differently, a way that the Lord originally intended. With the use of eight spiritual gifts purchased for us at the cross, we can do what He told Adam to do in the Garden and what we rarely hear from the nutrition authorities: eat freely.

INTRODUCTION

To begin, I think it is essential to establish several basic concepts to provide a fundamental framework from which to launch. First is that the Bible is the infallible Word of God, and the words written on its pages are indisputably right. The Bible tells us in 2 Timothy 3:16-17, "All Scripture is given by inspiration of God, and is profitable for doctrine, for reproof, for correction, for instruction in righteousness, that the man of God may be complete, thoroughly equipped for every good work." Additionally, the men who penned the Bible were guided and inspired by the Holy Spirit. Each word, from beginning to end, is intentional and instructional for you.

Second, is that Creation occurred. The Garden of Eden was an actual place. When Adam and Eve ate the forbidden fruit, sin and imperfection became part of our DNA. As a result, the relationship with God changed. We separated from Him both spiritually and physically.

Third, Jesus died on the cross and rose again three days later. His death paid our sin debt in full, and we are reconciled back into a personal relationship with God.

Finally, God is interested in and cares about our food. In Genesis 1:11, we read, "Then God said, 'Let the land produce vegetation: seed-bearing plants and trees on the land that bear fruit with seed in it, according to their various kinds.' And it was so." After the land produced per God's command, we read in verse 12 of the same chapter that He "saw that it was good." All of this was in preparation for Adam's much anticipated arrival. In Genesis 1:28, after Adam was created, God instructed him to be fruitful and multiply, and to rule over the animals created. After assigning Adam with responsibility, He then presents Adam with his very first gift. In verse 29, we read, "Then God said, 'I give you every seed-bearing plant on the face of the whole earth and every tree that has fruit and seed in it. They will be yours for food.'"

Research tells us most of the food in our supermarkets today did not exist a century ago. We are exposed to a food supply that has gotten out of control. Food is no longer simple or straightforward. Farmers can grow it. And scientists can create it. But they are not the same thing. We tend to define food today as something that we can consume by mouth, regardless of who made it or even how it was made. Dr. Mark Hyman challenges us to think about an interesting perspective. He says, "Think about it: if there is a health food section in the grocery store, what does that make the rest of the food sold there?" Well, that's food for thought, isn't it?

No matter how you view it, we are a food-centric society. Food is an integral part of our daily lives. And there are several conscious and unconscious decisions and choices we make regarding food every day. That said, food factors heavily into our weight loss or body composition goals, and our quest for health recovery or maintenance. It is typically the center of attention at all our celebrations, ceremonies, and family traditions. What ultimately rests on our meal plate on any given day is driven by what we permit ourselves to eat. Whether it is influenced by several factors that could include taste, convenience, comfort, or culture, typically, we get to make the decision.

In Genesis 2:8-9, we read "Now the Lord God had planted a garden in the east, in Eden; and there he put the man he had formed. The Lord God made all kinds of trees grow out of the ground — trees that were pleasing to the eye and good for food."

The Lord created and designed plants, the fruit of trees, and animals to be our food. Each of these were spoken into existence by the Creator Himself as a gift for man. So how then did food become such a complex topic? Since there's nothing we can add to the value of food, nor can we improve upon its health-giving capabilities, how can we really make what God made better? If anything, we have made it worse. Research now shows someone would have to eat five apples today to get the same nutritional value as an apple from the 1950s.

Food is a complex topic. If you were to talk about food with a group of friends, there would likely be little consensus on the right food to eat, how much to eat, how often to eat, and even when to eat. Much of the discussion would center on each person's successes and failures with diet goals, any recent research that they have conducted, as well as any health issues they may be experiencing. For example, some people are intolerant of gluten; therefore, they feel very strongly that gluten should be avoided. The same can be said for dairy, carbohydrates, saturated fat, high fructose corn syrup, and the like. People have differing opinions about what to eat and what not to eat. At any given moment, someone you know is doing Keto, while another is counting calories or macronutrients, while another is scarfing down fast food at least two times a day. Yet, another friend may be intermittent fasting. Each person can only offer opinions based on their personal experience, which is based on trial and error. With such disparity, trying to plan a meal together would be a nightmarish challenge!

Does the topic of food have to be so complicated and sophisticated? At least once, yet more likely on numerous occasions, every person has reached a point in their life where they feel like food is too hard to understand. And it is. Because we have made it so. That is probably the one unifying principle in this whole topic. It is the one experience we all have in common. It seems incredibly unfair to have to feed yourself every day and not know if you are doing it correctly or whether you are feeding yourself in the way best suited to your body's needs. Furthermore, your body's needs can and will change over the course of time. Is your focus weight loss? Cancer prevention? Cancer recovery? Diabetes?

Gluten Intolerance? Indigestion? All of these become significant factors in choosing the food you eat. Are you making decisions based on a lack of knowledge? Should you be required to know more? When is enough, enough? When eating right is a moving target, and the nutrition authorities keep changing their advice, it's natural to tire of the effort and throw your hands up in despair. You are justified in believing, "What does it matter anyway? No one knows the answers," while you order pizza delivery on speed- dial.

It requires a lot of brain energy to think about what to eat. Sometimes it feels good not to have to think about it at all. For this reason, we tend to eat the same foods. We buy the same groceries. We cook the same meals. The more routine we can make eating, the more comfortable we become. It frees up energy to focus on all the other things we must do every day. It is a vicious cycle. We've all been there, and there is no escape from it. We are bombarded with food advertisements and with diet programs to correct the consumption mistakes when our clothes start feeling a little tighter or when the number on the scale starts creeping upward. The ads will console you by telling you not to worry because it's not your fault. You just need their magic pill that burns off that unwanted fat while you sleep. Lucky for you, if you act now, you can get it for the low, low price of $19.99! Whether it's an over-the-counter medication, a weight loss supplement, or a prescription drug, the root of the problem is still there.

The relationship with food has become dysfunctional. The common way of thinking is that food is the enemy, and the reason people don't feel well. And it's no wonder! Most people feel abused by it. I was at lunch with some friends, and we were discussing food and the struggles they have with trying to decide what to eat. One of the friends presented an interesting perspective. She mentioned how one of her family members plans when they will eat ice cream because they know the next day, they will not feel well. Their stomach will bother them. They don't want to miss work, so they eat ice cream only on the weekend. What an interesting dynamic with food! We have all experienced the physical and emotional consequences of the cruel relationship. TV commercials even document the embarrassing scene. The creators of the advertisement portray slices of bacon or pizza, punching you or slapping you in the face while you are riding in the taxi on the way to your destination. You slide closer to the window, attempting to distance yourself from the one-sided food fight since you are physically unable to defend yourself. Instead of being able to prepare for the meeting you are headed to, you are helplessly victimized by your previous meal. All of this takes place while the other passengers in the vehicle look on helplessly but with pity and horror as you have no choice but to endure each greasy blow. Sadly, we can all relate to this scenario. While we have probably never been physically assaulted by a slice of pizza, our stomach rumblings, or even the inadvertent belch or worse (gasp!), let people around us know that our food didn't agree with us. That there is a fight-a'brewin' down below. The worst part of it all is that you are the one who selected the food and then ate it!

We have turned over the responsibility of nourishing

ourselves to the food industry, government, and the person working the drive-thru window of our favorite fast-food chain. Because the topic of food is so difficult to navigate and requires too much energy to research, it's just easier to trust others to make the decisions. Admittedly, we are not interested in the nutrition it offers. Instead, we are more interested in the convenience the industry is selling. The government and the food industry wouldn't have any other interest in food other than your health and nourishment, right? According to Michael Moss, the food industry is competing over something called "stomach share." It is all about profit. "Stomach share" is the "amount of digestive space that any one company's brand can grab from the competition." It is how they measure your dollars. The CEO's of the big food companies try "to get a larger share of what people [eat]." Even though the CEO's of America's largest food companies were made aware of their contribution to the obesity epidemic, reducing the sugar or addictive quality could mean a considerable loss of "stomach share." After being presented with the incriminating facts, Stephen Sanger, head of General Mills at the time, said, "Don't talk to me about nutrition. Talk to me about taste, and if this stuff tastes better, don't run around trying to sell stuff that doesn't taste good."

According to the 2019 film, *The Food That Built America*, "Today, the food industry drives more than one-fifth of the U. S. economy ... it fuels one in four American jobs ... and generates more than 5 billion dollars ... a day." Most Americans rely on other people to feed them.

For many, having to eat is like repeatedly having to

engage in the same argument several times a day. You know you must interact, but it's not going to end well. And you don't know how to fix it. But what choice do you have? How else are you supposed to nourish yourself? The dysfunction is so commonplace that we don't even see it anymore. On any given day, most people probably have more Tums in their bag than chewing gum. The dysfunction is painfully real, and it's normal. It can take on many forms, such as indigestion, heartburn, or that all-too-familiar cramping in your stomach after you eat. Dysfunction can manifest as a lack of energy, feeling tired, or having the 3:00 p.m. crash. There's no shame in admitting that you are a sugar addict because everyone else you know is too. It is all abuse. All we can do is try to minimize the damage. Now, let me be clear. I am not in any way saying that medical attention and the use of prescription medications are wrong. What I am saying is that we tend to view them as the only answer. Food is an unavoidable evil that will hurt you but take this pill to make the pain go away. The vicious cycle continues.

Considering where we are today, it's worth looking into where food came from and how the dysfunctional relationship began. As Bible-believing Christians, we have a choice. It is time to take a stand and believe what the Bible tells us about our relationship to food. But most Christians have no idea what the Bible says. Without even realizing it, we have substituted the relationship with Jesus for our relationship with food.

Remember, based on the information in Genesis, the first mention of food was that of a source of enjoyment for Adam.

It was a gift. God said it was good. It was perfectly designed for man's body and for man's consumption. When Adam arrived in the Garden, there were no menus. There were no food scales, nor were there any dietary guidelines. There weren't even mirrors so that Eve could see if her hips were getting too big because she ate too many mangos. Adam gave no thought about the nutritional makeup of his food or where he could find it. Because it was God's provision for His much-anticipated guest, Adam's greatest concern was whether he was going to eat the delicious, juicy pineapple or taste a fruit that he had never had before. Either way, he gave no thought to whether it would be delicious, nutritious, and good for his body because everything was. It was exactly what God told him. It was pleasing to the eye and good for food. He could eat freely.

Wouldn't it be nice to get back to that? To be able to enjoy what you eat? To not have to worry whether you have made the right choice? Because the Fall of Man happened in the Garden when they ate the forbidden fruit, it separated them and us from God. The cross was necessary to reestablish the intimate relationship with God. Understanding the Garden of Eden and the Cross together, I believe that, for the Christian, our relationship with food changed. Sin changed our relationship with God and with food for the worse. The cross fixed it. As Christians, we don't live it because we don't know it. While the cross provided us a way back to God as well as prevented us from being eternally separated from Him, it also changed the Christian's relationship with the first gift God gave man: food. We will see in this book that, after the Garden, God gave us eight additional gifts that we can use in our relationship to food: grace, righteousness, faith, peace, wisdom, thanksgiving, seeds, and communion.

The relationship we have with food has gotten way off course. Most people don't trust that they are making the right choice because of the conflicting opinions and advice coming from authoritative sources such as the government and doctors. No matter what you do, there is a nagging thought that you can always do better. I hope that if we can return to a better understanding of what food originally was and how the Lord designed for us to eat it, with the use of the additional gifts, there will be a freedom to enjoy God's first gift. We will be better able to weed through all the science and diet trends to find a relationship with food that the Lord initially intended for each of us. If food is one of the original gifts provided in the Garden of Eden, how did it become such a source of frustration, confusion, sickness, and disease? With all the information that I have gathered from my years studying nutrition as well as my familiarity with the Bible, I hope to find clarity and share it with you.

Arguably, everyone wants to feel well. Everyone would like unlimited energy. Everyone would also like not to have to worry about food. Living this way is an extreme departure from the Garden of Eden. God created food for man to enjoy.

I believe that the Bible is the greatest nutritional manual ever written. Our Creator wrote it as a guidebook for us to live a victorious life. And food is a necessary part of that equation. Without food, we will die. But with the food we are eating today, many people are dying. Our bodies are designed to function on food. Therefore, it would make sense that a loving Father who sent His Son to reconcile us to Him and pay the sin debt in full would leave no stone unturned. The crucifixion corrected every aspect of what sin disrupted. And food is part of that.

This book's intent is to be used as a guidebook to help you develop a greater understanding of who you are and what you have because of the cross. The following chapters will each address a gift and how it relates to your relationship with food. The result will be a greater understanding of how the cross not only changed our spiritual condition; it changed our relationship to food as well.

Psalm 34:8 "Taste and see that the Lord is good."

CHAPTER 1

CONCEPT INTRO AND THE GARDEN

In this section of the book, we will be discussing the two most pivotal events of the Christian faith: The Garden of Eden and the Crucifixion. Without the main sin event in the Garden, there would have been no need for the Crucifixion. However, without the Crucifixion, we would each have to pay for and live with the fatal consequences of the original sin in the Garden. As we discussed in the Introduction, food was God's unique gift to Adam. As such, we can safely assume that food is something incredibly special to our Creator. Welcoming His guest into the Garden, God could have given Adam a hand-picked bouquet of beautiful flowers, or He could have arranged for the most magnificent aerial light show. He could have even choreographed an animal-packed, wildly entertaining musical number that would have rivaled the "Be Our Guest" performance in Disney's movie "Beauty and the Beast." When you think about it, God could have created anything to welcome Adam into the Garden. But a vital component of the welcome packet was food. He wanted food to be part of Adam's enjoyment. He designed Adam's body to use the food. And He gave Adam the freedom to eat it. Comparatively speaking, part of our struggle today is the loss of this enjoyment and freedom.

The freedom to eat the food in the Garden came with a command to not eat of the Tree of the Knowledge of Good and Evil. Ironically, with the restriction, this is the height of freedom. The Lord laid out the parameters. Loosely paraphrased, the Lord told Adam to eat anything and everything except this one thing. I repeat, one thing. We can all relate to this but on a grander scale. Today, we have it somewhat reversed. When anyone talks of dieting, they typically list all the foods they can no longer eat. Their perspective becomes focused on the limitations or what foods we need to avoid. Whenever there are so many limits, it doesn't feel like freedom because it's not. We are accustomed to living under eating and dieting rules. There is all this food available, but you can't partake. You can't eat carbs. You can't eat bacon. You can't eat fat. You can't eat any more than a certain number of calories. You get the picture.

Admittedly, there have been instances in my past when I have said, "I wish I didn't have to think about food. I wish I could just take a pill and move on with my day." To many people, that would be a perfect world. To others, they would miss the experience of eating. It's energy-draining and time consuming to have to think about what to eat or what not to eat, the calories or the macronutrients, or what food can be combined efficiently with another. I want simplicity. Just give me the pill, please!

But in the perfect world of the Garden, the Lord planned out every detail that man would need. The Garden consisted of "every tree ... that is pleasant to the sight and good for food." There was the Tree of Life and the Tree of the Knowledge of Good and Evil. There was a river, a woman, and every beast of the field and every bird of the air. Also, the Lord would walk through the Garden, providing and enjoying the fellowship and companionship with the First Couple. The Garden was the place of man's intimate relationship with the Lord. Adam and Eve both had a positive relationship with food because they had a positive relationship with God.

I'm not sure why the Tree of the Knowledge of Good and Evil was in the Garden. Knowing that answer is beyond my pay grade and the scope of this book. I recently heard a preacher say that the tree was there because God wanted to give man free will. God didn't create robots. He wanted Adam to want to be in the relationship. When Adam ate the fruit, he was choosing the fruit over God. But for our purposes, what we need to know is that eating of that one tree would and did result in death. Letting my imagination wander a bit, I wonder what type of fruit did the Tree of the Knowledge of Good and Evil produce. Could you get that fruit on another tree, or was that the only source? Several artists have depicted the pivotal scene with Eve pulling or having already pulled an apple from the tree. In 1512,

Michelangelo adorned the ceiling of the Sistine Chapel with The Fall and Expulsion from Garden of Eden. Rubens captures the moment in his 1628–1629 painting entitled The Fall of Man. For whatever reason, the Bible doesn't explicitly provide us with that fruit identification. Based on artist renditions, we commonly refer to the fruit as an apple.

From a sensory perspective, imagine the sweet, fruity smell of the air in the Garden. The combination of the distinct scent of peaches, pineapples, and apples, among other delectable options. The fruit was never mealy, mushy, or moldy. You didn't have to battle fruit flies. The fruit was always at the peak sweetness and juiciness. Each fruit was brilliantly and vibrantly colored in the appropriately and lovingly designed hues. There couldn't be any blemishes or worms to be pleasing to the sight. There were orchards and more orchards beautifully displayed with branches bending under the weight of the bounty. Remember the story of the Israelite spies entering the Promised Land in Numbers 13:23? It took two men to carry the bunch of grapes! Imagine what they looked like in the Garden. Sadly, we will never know, but it is kind of exciting to think about. What we do know is that they were perfect and perfectly suited for Adam. Just focusing on the fruit in the Garden provides us with a reference of the generosity and provision of a loving God.

God deemed the food good. I can only imagine the experience of eating perfect food. Especially since today, we tend to struggle with enjoying our food. If it is something we enjoy, often we feel guilty that we do. Typically, the enjoyment comes from eating something that is not good for us or is laden with salt or sugar. Sadly, that is by the design of the food industry. There aren't many people who can say they enjoy an apple over their favorite candy bar. Yet, we were designed to enjoy our food. The food industry has researched and capitalized on the brain's response to foods such as sugar, salt, and fat. In Michael Moss's book *Salt, Sugar, Fat: How the Food Giants Hooked Us*, the author describes how scientists, chemists, and researchers, hired by the food industry leaders, studied a human's response to certain foods. They determined the perfect combination of ingredients, including chemicals, to provide the ideal "mouth feel," and "bliss point," to keep you coming back for more. Our ability to enjoy food has been manipulated into addiction, dependency, and struggle.

Based on Adam's relationship to food in the Garden, we see that we were designed to enjoy the look, the feel, and the taste of food, making this a healthy relationship. Being that our design hasn't changed, we should still be able to enjoy this healthy relationship. But sadly, we don't live in the Garden of Eden.

That now brings us to the rest of the story. As ominous music begins to play, you know that something terrible is about to happen. And it does. The serpent approaches Eve.

There are no introductions. There are no how-do-you-dos. The serpent is on a mission. Right out of the gate the serpent asks Eve a simple question: "Did God say, 'You must not eat from any tree in the garden?'" Eve replies "We may eat fruit from the trees in the garden, but God did say, 'You must not eat fruit from the tree that is in the middle of the garden, and you must not touch it, or you will die.'" No, no, no! God never said anything about touching the fruit! At that moment, the serpent knew he had her because she wasn't clear on what God had said. Either taking away or adding to His words can have the same destructive and confusing effect. If only she confidently knew what God had said, maybe the ending would have been vastly different! I have often thought that when I get to Heaven, I'm going to find Eve and ask her why she ate the forbidden food. Didn't she realize she had so many other options? Why did she feel the need to eat that fruit? Then I realize how many times I have eaten something I knew I shouldn't. So, maybe I'll just leave it at "Hey Eve. Nice to meet you."

Arguably, this is the condition we as Christians are in today. What does God's Word say about food? Most people could not tell you. They simply don't know. They mention something about gluttony or maybe even the Daniel fast, but what about the actual topic of food? When we don't know what God says, we leave ourselves open to distraction and the opportunity to be misled by others who we believe are in authority. Just like with Eve, there are dire consequences to not knowing.

Now, back to the story. The serpent replies, "You will not certainly die. For God knows that when you eat from it, your eyes will be opened, and you will be like God, knowing good and evil."

The woman then looked at the tempting fruit. It met the criteria: it was good for food and pleasing to the eye. But she added a quality that God never used to describe food. In

Genesis 3:6 we read, "When the woman saw that the fruit of the tree was ... also desirable for gaining wisdom, she took some and ate it." The serpent convinced the woman that God was withholding something from her. In the perfect Garden environment, she believed that she needed something more. Eve took the fateful bite and forever altered the course of humanity. The enemy convinced Eve that the food she was instructed not to eat would provide her with something she was missing. As a result, sin entered the world with all its consequences, including separation from God. It also included death, both physically and spiritually.

If only Eve had known God's instructions and been able to recognize the serpent for who he was. The story would be much different. Thankfully, we have the benefit of Eve's hindsight.

I know this is basic Bible stuff. Often, new Christians learn the story of the Garden of Eden in Sunday School. But, in looking deeper from a nutritional perspective, at the precise moment that sin entered the Garden, Adam and Eve's relationship to food changed as well, again, both physically and spiritually.

Physically, God punished Adam for his involvement by cursing the ground from which the food grew. "Through painful toil, you will eat food from it." That is about as physical as you can get. But that is not all. "By the sweat of your brow, you will eat your food." What a departure from having free and unlimited access to the most varied produce department anyone would ever know! It is interesting to note that the use of the word "food" here in this verse is translated "bread" in the Hebrew language. The word is *lechem*. You can't pick bread from a tree. You must grow the grain, harvest, sift, mix it, and knead it, all before consuming it. That takes planning, time, and a lot of effort.

Adam's punishment is the first time that the word food/bread or *lechem* is used in the Bible. According to Jewish wisdom, there is a significance to the first mention of a word. It indicates something that we should pay attention to. All previous and original references to food in Genesis refer to the Hebrew word *okla*, which simply means "food, what is consumed" or *makal* in the Hebrew, which means "something to eat, food or fruit."

Because I am kind of a word nerd, I found it interesting that another variation of the Hebrew word *lechem* is *laham*, as used in Adam's punishment is "battle or war." Has anyone ever heard reference to the "Battle of the Bulge?" in connection with weight loss, or because of health care costs, we need to wage "War on Obesity?" How many times have you heard of someone's personal battle with an eating disorder? These are dysfunctional relationships to food arguably part of the sin punishment.

There is no doubt that Adam's days of convenience food were over. From that point on, if he was going to eat, he had to work for it. It's no coincidence that our attempt to reinstitute convenience typically involves food that is not good for us. We have fast food drive-thrus. We have microwaves. We have processed, precooked, or boxed meals. For a food to sit on a shelf for weeks or months without spoiling, that product must be highly preserved. According to factmyth.com,

Thomas DeMichele researched the urban legend that a Hostess Twinkie will never go bad. The author reports, "According to "Twinkie, Deconstructed" by Steve Ettlinger, a Twinkie can last up to 30 years ... but it will be hard and brittle." He continues, "The 'sell-by' shelf life of a Twinkie is 45 days." Can you imagine what an orange would look like after 45 days?

My niece, nephew, and I bought a McDonald's Happy Meal with cheese on my niece's birthday ten years ago. We also purchased a Burger King Kids Meal two months later on my nephew's birthday.

To date, I still have both meals sitting in my pantry. They have never been refrigerated. They both contain cheese and bread, which never molded. Nor did they ever attract ants, thankfully. The only attention the Burger King meal has received since the time of purchase is that I needed to put the food into a new paper bag because the original became oily. I also needed to place the French fries with their original paper sleeve into a plastic zip-top bag due to the grease leaking out of the package. Other than that, both meals look disturbingly like the day I bought them. It doesn't really fit the food definition, but I digress.

Based on the bread/battle terminology, I think it is safe to say that part of Adam's punishment in the Garden would be a continued struggle with food. There is a physical desire to eat more than we need and to eat what tastes good even though it may not be good for us. Sadly, most people in this country are overfed and undernourished. The food industry, the diet food industry, and the medical industry have all capitalized on this. Please don't think that I am assigning ulterior motives to all parties. But they have recognized a need and are benefitting from it.

A point worth noting is that every time Adam makes bread, it is a painful reminder of the one act of sin they committed in the Garden. It is no different today. Food is incredibly powerful, evoking memories and prompting emotions, both good and bad.

In John 6:35, Jesus refers to Himself as the "Bread of Life." Isn't that beautiful? Immediately following the sin, buried within the punishment, was the remediation of that punishment: Jesus. In verse 28, the disciples asked Jesus, "What must we do to do the works that God requires?" Jesus answers by telling them, "The work of God is this: to believe in the one He has sent." In other words, we simply believe in Jesus. Needing a sign to believe, the disciples recalled how God gave their ancestors "bread from heaven to eat." They were referring to the manna that was provided every day so they wouldn't starve while wandering out in the Wilderness. But Jesus then says something unexpected to His disciples. He tells them, "My Father gives you the true bread from Heaven. For the bread of God is the bread that comes down from heaven and gives life to the world." Jesus then declares, "I am the bread of life." In verse 51, we read, "I am the living bread that came down from Heaven. Whoever eats this bread will live forever. This bread is my flesh, which I will give for the life of the world."

We read in His Word that "Man does not live by bread alone. But by every word that proceeds from the mouth of the

Lord." At the time of the expulsion from the Garden, all Adam had was bread. Think about that statement, with the benefit of hindsight. For the time being, Adam would have to work for his food. It was up to him alone. He didn't realize that God had already promised the answer: Jesus, the Bread of Life. Even though Adam was separated from God because of the sin, God was forecasting the way to reinstitute the relationship. His name is Jesus. You see, Adam and Eve were not the only ones who lost something that day. God did too. He lost fellowship. Immediately, He used Adam's food to represent the way back to Him. Here we can see that there is a physical and spiritual element to food.

According to Rabbi Daniel Lapin, food has a spiritual dimension. He teaches, "Just as humans are both physical and spiritual, so is food." We can see the dichotomy in the Garden. As soon as Eve ate the forbidden physical fruit, she introduced spiritual death for which the cross would be required.

There is a higher dimension to food than what we learn in the church. Christians are functioning in this world at a significant disadvantage. They don't know about the positive relationship they can have with food. In the Garden, we lost it. At the cross, we got it back.

CHAPTER 2

THE CROSS

Thank goodness for the Crucifixion. If Jesus had never died on the cross, we would be responsible for our sin debt. A debt each of us is ill-equipped to pay. The very moment Adam and Eve ate the forbidden fruit, and as the serpent advertised would happen, their eyes were opened. They were now aware of spiritual things they previously knew nothing about. The resulting physical and spiritual separation was immediate. But notice in Genesis 3:10, we read that Adam hid from God. He initiated the physical separation while God was looking for him. Then in verse 23 of the same chapter, we learn that "the Lord God banished" them from the Garden.

For a man to interact with God, certain restrictions or protections had to occur. Otherwise, man would die simply because, in man's sin state, he cannot live in the presence of a perfect, sinless God. For example, while Moses was receiving the Ten Commandments, if an Israelite touched Mount Sinai, where God was, they would immediately die. The Bible tells of many instances where a man was not permitted to see God's face. When God cut the covenant between Himself and Abraham, He caused Abraham to fall asleep to protect him from seeing God. We also see in the Old Testament that Moses was not permitted to see God's face. He had to hide in the cleft of a rock to shield himself from God's glory. When the Israelites were led through the Wilderness, they were only permitted to see God's back. He led them by a cloud during the day and a pillar of fire at night, but always in front of them. God's holiness is so powerful and so demanding that, in man's sinful state, he cannot survive in His presence. The chasm between our sin and God's perfection was immeasurable and fatal. There was nothing man could do to make up the difference. All seemed lost until the cross. Jesus took on all our sins, sicknesses, and diseases requiring God to turn His back on His Son. Because of the cross, there will never be a need for God to turn His back to us. We will always see His face. We can boldly declare, "Lord, let your face shine upon us."

Before the cross, when the priests entered the temple, they had to spiritually and physically cleanse; otherwise, they would be struck dead. Approaching or being in the presence of a perfect, holy God couldn't be taken lightly. It could and would cost you your life. But after Jesus paid the sin debt, the veil was torn so we "can boldly come to the throne of grace." In Mark 15:38, we read the curtain of the temple was torn in two. This signified that there was no more separation between God and man. The relationship with God was restored, and we can now approach God in Jesus's righteousness and not our imperfection. When we put on the robe of righteousness, God doesn't see our sin. He only sees the precious blood of His Son, who paid the debt in full.

Interestingly, the little phrase "in full" is critical to our understanding of the Christian's relationship to food. Since Jesus is considered the Second Adam, the payment for our sin "in full" means that no consequence of the sin debt Adam incurred remains.

While Genesis chapter 3 provides a specific breakdown of the punishment specific to the serpent, Eve, and Adam, there were changes that took place before the penalty phase.

First, there is separation. Adam instinctively felt the inherent need to hide from God. He initiated the separation. It was temporary. He would eventually come out from behind the tree. It wasn't until the penalty dispensation that the separation became God-imposed and permanent.

There was also fear. The first instance fear is mentioned anywhere in the Bible occurred in verse 10 when Adam admitted to God that he was afraid because he was naked. In other words, Adam recognized that he was unprotected and vulnerable. Up until this moment, Adam had nothing to be afraid of and was unfamiliar with the emotion of fear.

Beginning with Genesis 3:14, the consequences of eating the forbidden fruit were doled out to each guilty party. God began with the serpent, followed by the woman, then the man. Notably, for our purposes here, Adam's consequences pertain to food. Now, God told Adam when He instructed him not to eat of the tree, that if "you eat from it; you will certainly die." So, according to God's Word, the moment they ate of the fruit, death entered their world. When God addressed Adam's punishment, there was a reference to mortality: "through painful toil, you will eat food [from the ground] all the days of your life" and "By the sweat of your brow, you will eat your food until you return to the ground ... to dust, you will return."

So here we have all that death entails. Eating the fruit meant that Adam would surely die. God was not talking only about the moment that the heart stops beating. There are slow, protracted stages of death that we see every day, such as sickness, disease, loss of energy, and aches and pains. These are a part of life that we tend to tolerate or accept as normal under the process of "aging."

Additionally, the relationship to food changed drastically. Adam now had to plan and work for it. Also, the stress associated with being afraid and the radical lifestyle change causes a biological response in the body that changes how that body processes food. Under stress, or preferably in a fight or flight condition, digestive functions diminish, and the nervous system switches from parasympathetic to sympathetic, or in other words, from rest to fight or flight. This switch changes the body's reaction to food. Imagine the chronic stress Adam was initially under trying to figure out how to feed himself and his family. He didn't have a recipe book from the Garden library or a collection of family favorites from Eve's mother and grandmother. He had to figure it out while his stomach was growling, and the kids were complaining. For our purposes today, the impact of stress is essential to mention. Many people are under the impression that all you need to do is eat the right diet. But what if your body is unable to break down the perfect diet because we are so chronically stressed, and digestion has become compromised? We will save that topic for later. So why are Christians struggling with food issues and sickness? If sickness and working for food are the consequence of sin, as described in the previous chapter, and Jesus paid the sin debt in full, then shouldn't there no longer be any lingering consequences? Or are they the consequences we tolerate or believe are just a normal part of life? The Bible tells us that we are in the world, not of the world. So, shouldn't there be a noticeable difference in a Christian's relationship to food?

Several years ago, I had one of those a-ha moments. I started to research the broader application of the crucifixion to my life. I learned the crucifixion didn't just occur on the cross. There were several stages to Jesus' death, each of which holds their significance and application to the Christian life. It began with the Lord's Supper. The disciples were attempting to find a location to hold the traditional Passover Supper on the first day of the Festival of Unleavened Bread. According to Mark 14:17-18, "When evening came, Jesus arrived with the Twelve. While they were reclining at the table eating, he said, 'Truly I tell you, one of you will betray me – one who is eating with me.'" In verses 22 through 24, "Jesus took bread, and when he had given thanks, he broke it and gave it to his disciples, saying, 'Take it; this is my body.' Then he took a cup, and when he had given thanks, he gave it to them, and they all drank from it. 'This is my blood of the covenant, which is poured out for many,' he said to them."

The Passover Supper is a traditional Jewish celebration. When the Israelites were enslaved in Egypt, God instructed Moses to approach Pharaoh with the message, "Let my people go." Despite several devastating plagues from the Lord, Pharaoh refused. The final motivation was the Lord killing the firstborn of every "people and animal" in Egypt who failed to apply the blood of a spotless lamb on their doorpost. They were instructed to apply the blood to the top and sides of the doorframe. I have heard it preached that the blood was applied in the shape of a cross. In Exodus 12:23, we read in part, "the Lord ... will see the blood ... and will pass over that doorway, and he will not permit the destroyer to enter your houses and strike you down." The Israelite slaves were immediately released. Notice the difference the blood made. Among all the inhabitants of Egypt, some people were exempt from the consequences. In other words, they were in Egypt, but not of Egypt, when the blood protected them. This protection was a foreshadowing of the protective, consequence changing blood of Jesus.

After the Lord's Supper, the party moved to the Garden of Gethsemane. While Jesus prayed, He sweat drops of blood. Luke 22:44 tells us, "And being in anguish, he prayed more earnestly, and his sweat was like drops of blood falling to the ground." Wow! Jesus's blood is powerful to cleanse sin, right? And the ground was cursed because of sin? Then wouldn't it stand to reason that the curse of the land was removed with one drop of His blood? Let's revisit the cursing of the ground. The ground had already been cursed as part of Adam's punishment. God commanded it to produce weeds and thorns. God cursed the ground again because of Cain killing his brother Abel. In Genesis 4:12, God tells Cain, "When you work the ground, it will no longer yield its crops for you." This curse, hampering the ability to eat, was specifically for Cain. But it shows that God has the power to control the ground. After the Flood, when God is talking to Noah, He doesn't mention that the original curse is lifted. In Genesis 8:21, God tells Noah, "Never again will I curse the ground because of humans, even though every inclination of the human heart is evil from childhood." This promise to Noah confused me. The Flood wiped everyone and everything off the face of the earth except Noah and his family, along with a male and female pair of every animal. So, if the cursed ground is a consequence of the original sin, then the shedding of Jesus's blood in the Garden of Gethsemane would be the only remedy to lift the curse.

Next, Jesus is arrested, tried, and found guilty. He is taken to the whipping post and beaten. This location is significant because this is where Jesus obtained the necessary stripes to fulfill the prophetic words of Isaiah 53:5, "By His stripes, we are healed." Jesus then carries His cross to Golgotha, "the place of the skull," where He was eventually crucified. During this slow and agonizing experience, according to the prophecy in Isaiah 53:4, "Surely he took up our pain and bore our suffering, yet we considered Him punished by God. ... But he was pierced for our transgressions, he was crushed for our iniquities." When all the consequences of the sin from the Garden of Eden are paid for by His perfect, sinless blood, Jesus cries, "It is finished." At that point, the sin debt was paid in full. And part of the sin debt was a changed relationship to food. Since the payment is in full, then the Crucifixion changed our relationship to food as well.

CHAPTER 3

PREMISE

In 1948, Winston Churchill said, "Those who fail to learn from history are condemned to repeat it." Churchill was quoting a gentleman by the name of George Santayana, who, in 1905, said: "Those who cannot remember the past are condemned to repeat it." While there are subtle differences between the two quotes, the point remains and is worth addressing here: knowing history is essential to not repeat past mistakes. Typically, when we think of history, we think of American history and its leading events, which include slavery, women's right to vote, world wars, innovations, and even dark times we want to preclude from ever occurring again. But what about a Christian's history? The key events in that timeline include the Garden of Eden and the Crucifixion.

We need to understand how the serpent assisted Eve in eating the forbidden fruit. She presumably walked past the

Tree of the Knowledge of Good and Evil on numerous occasions with no thought of ever approaching it. However, the basis of the deception wasn't that the fruit would taste better than others. Instead, it was that if she ate the fruit, she "would be like God, knowing good and evil." Because she didn't know what God had said, she easily believed the serpent. The serpent never told her to eat the fruit, nor did he force it down her throat. He simply took advantage of her ignorance. He asked her, "Did God really say ...?" He subtly and strategically led her down a path she wasn't even aware she was traveling. Because the serpent had been cast out of Heaven, he was angry and was calculating his revenge. Eve fell for the deception by the one whose only motivation was and is to "kill, steal, and destroy."

Since the serpent was separated from God, he wanted Adam and Eve separated too. If the enemy can keep us separated from God, then we are left vulnerable as prime targets. He activated his plan by causing Eve doubt when it came to her food. The enemy is a one-trick pony. What he has done in the past, he will do again. If he can keep us focused on our relationship with food, if he can create enough confusion or cause just enough doubt to make the topic of food seem too complicated, then he leaves us distracted from the real answer: Jesus. You see, it is not about food at all. It's about the relationship with God.

This relationship leads me to an essential question: Do you know what God says about food? If someone were to challenge you the way the serpent did Eve, would you be able to take a definitive stance on your belief? Eve's uncertainty about God's instructions regarding food cost her, and humanity, everything.

We know about the Garden. We have read the story countless times. But do we really know about it? Or are we just familiar with the story? Granted, it was a long time ago, and no one will ever live in the perfect utopia of the Garden of Eden, so why does it matter? Why is it so crucial to our relationship with food today?

Similarly, we know about the cross. We are familiar with the story. We see it portrayed on cable television in the movie The Passion of the Christ at Easter and in the church Christmas pageant every December. But do we know about it? Why is it so crucial to our relationship with food today?

We have assigned food power and control over our lives that we don't recognize or understand. We attribute most ills or adverse health consequences to what we have or have not eaten. We think about food ... often. Health authorities instruct us to think about food. We are told to eat a certain way. We are given so many options that it's difficult to decipher. Yet ultimately, what we put in our mouth is up to us individually. No one shoves the food in our mouth. We have free will; we have the privilege to make choices. Just like in the Garden, Adam and Eve had the opportunity to eat or not to eat from the forbidden tree. But their choice had to be rooted in knowledge. Without knowledge of the truth to galvanize our decisions, we are easily confused and, at times, deceived.

Food is an integral part of our lives. It is a necessity. Without food, we would eventually die. Food is everywhere.

It is in your refrigerator, cabinets, pantries, secret stashes, grocery stores, convenience stores, pharmacies, gas stations, restaurants, fast food chains, vending machines, desk drawer, concession stands, church socials, holiday parties, family events, celebrations, funerals, social events with friends, amusement parks, shopping malls, hospitals, and school and corporate cafeterias. You can't go anywhere without food being provided or offered. So, because of its ubiquity, we need to have a grasp on our relationship with it.

Arguably the most significant and impactful event that ever took place for the Christian was the Crucifixion. This one event changed the course of the Christian's life and death forever. The Crucifixion is not just about our salvation from eternal damnation. Focusing only on the spiritual benefits of the cross doesn't take full advantage of Jesus's death; it doesn't adequately describe what the blood of Jesus bought back for us. Yes, it paid the sin debt in full. Yet, part of the sin debt was a changed relationship to food. Adam had to work for it. It was no longer readily accessible or convenient. The ground from which the food would grow was cursed. Death and all its derivatives were introduced and ultimately experienced by every person born after Adam and Eve. Their DNA changed at that very moment. Their genetic makeup now included sin. When God created food for Adam, it was for a man whose DNA was without sin. With a sinful DNA, arguably, the relationship to food changed. In 2 Corinthians 5:17, we are told: "Therefore if any man be in Christ, he is a new creature: old things are passed away; behold, all things become new." In a relationship with Jesus, a change takes place. The Christian's DNA is no longer stained with sin. After the cross, a Christian's DNA can respond to God-designed food just like Adam did. Even science is coming to grips with this fact. Our DNA responds to everything we eat. Each meal programs our genes with messages of health or sickness.

Epigenetics is a scientific study of environmental factors that influence gene expression. Those factors can include toxins and a person's diet. In other words, genes can be turned on or off based on what a person eats. The person's DNA structure doesn't change. The genetic makeup inherited from the parents is still there. Instead, the DNA expression can be regulated. From a scientific and nutritional standpoint, we see how food can influence our genetic makeup creating an environment for health or sickness. For the Christian, who is a new creature because of the cross, the DNA expression and relationship to food can go even deeper. Because of our genetic uniqueness, your Creator knows best the food you should eat. Alan Aragon, a nutrition researcher and educator states, "Every meal is ... a short-term investment in how you feel and perform, a mid-term investment in how you look, and a long-term investment in your freedom from disease."

Can we change the fact that we must work for our food? No. Can we change how food manufacturers are offering non-food items? No. In our quest to reinstate convenience, we buy processed, packaged foods. The food industry does not sell food. Admittedly, they sell convenience. We consume food that contains more preservatives and synthetic ingredients than we can pronounce. According to Dr. Mark Hyman,

"The food industry sells products scientifically proven to kill more people than cigarettes." Dr. Timothy Weeks states, "We have a healthcare system that cares nothing about food and a food system that cares nothing about health." We are not eating food anymore. We are eating a substance that is considered food based on a loose definition, but really, it is just a food-like substance.

Food, or better yet, putting something edible in our mouth, has become a reward. We don't just like food; we love it. We crave it. We love how it tastes. We love how it makes us feel. But our relationship with food continues to get more dysfunctional.

Our food comes with environmental concerns such as the use of Roundup, contaminated water, chlorine, pesticides, and the resulting nutrient depletion in the topsoil. Sadly, produce grown today contains minimal amounts of nutrients than it did 50 years ago. Often, after people eat, they feel bad. They experience heartburn. Their stomachs hurt. They are allergic to many of the ingredients. People are developing and battling eating disorders. Many are continually cycling through one diet to the next with the hopes of losing the weight. Typically, one of the first questions asked to a person in a health crisis is, "What have you been eating?" And part of the prescription is, "You need to change your diet." We simultaneously see food as both the problem and the answer.

Right after college, I began going to the gym and lifting weights. I didn't know much about resistance training at that time, but I had dabbled in it since the seventh grade. Carving out the time after work, I was very consistent. I even began going to the gym at 5:00 every morning. I loved it. The next time that I went for an annual checkup, the number on the scale had increased by a few pounds. I never weighed myself. I didn't even own a scale. My clothes didn't fit any differently, but my muscle mass had increased. I remember a time when my boyfriend introduced me to a friend of his. We had been out to dinner, and I was wearing a sleeveless top. After the introductions and before the obligatory "Nice to meet you," the friend exclaimed, "Wow, look at those guns!" I had been consistent with my workouts, and, admittedly, I was quite proud.

After reviewing my chart, the doctor looked at me and said, "You have gained weight since the last time you were here. You are on your way to developing a weight problem. Lay off the pizza." He stood up from his chair and exited the examination room. I was stunned. I could feel the tears beginning to sting my eyes. I had been so diligent about going to the gym. My diet wasn't bad, nor was it perfect. That advice from an uninformed, ignorant medical authority pushed me into a strict, dangerously rigid eating plan. I only ate egg whites and spinach for breakfast. I ate salads for lunch and then had a small dinner. I had to lose the exact number of pounds I had inadvertently gained in that year. Anytime I felt like I could relax my diet, I would recall the feeling I had when that doctor spoke those words to me. The problem was that I was still lifting weights. Adhering to the diet, it didn't take long for me to stop feeling energetic enough to go work out. I was simply running out of energy. My body was reducing my energy output to protect me. I was getting sick more often and catching just about every cough or cold that my co-workers decided to bring to the office. My body couldn't function with the little amount I was eating. But all that mattered was the number on the scale. If the doctor said my food was the problem, then, in my mind, the solution was to stop eating it.

I had my first knee surgery during my senior year in high school. I was devastated because it knocked me out of my final year of softball. As part of my rehab, my parents bought me a cross-country skiing machine. I loved that machine. I didn't care so much about the knee strengthening benefits. It was the 600 calories that I burned in a 30-minute workout. My way of thinking at that time was, if 30 minutes is good, then an hour must be even better! So, with extraordinarily little food in my system, I jumped on that machine every day. I was abiding by the popular rule: eat less, exercise more! One afternoon, after finishing my "knee rehab," I stopped by the kitchen to talk with my mom while she cooked dinner. While she was talking, I began to feel lightheaded with a strange underwater ringing in my ears. The black spots floating in front of my face were multiplying and beginning to hinder my vision. I grabbed the back of the chair in time before my knees buckled. My mom could see that something was wrong. She immediately sat me down in the chair and gave me something to eat. I was upset because I knew that the moment I ate, I negated all the benefits of "knee rehab."

I have always had a fascination with food. This fascination is especially ironic because I was still a picky eater. For example, I don't care for mashed potatoes because of the texture. I don't eat butter beans because, when I was a child, I thought they were hairy inside. I also think tomatoes smell like body odor. I know. It doesn't make sense. Having to fix meals for six people every day, I'm sure my food pickiness was a lot of fun for my mother.

Based on what I've been taught, food holds the key to our health successes or challenges. This teaching reminds me of the multiple variations of the same quote that states, "The greatest form of learning is unlearning." I realized this when I began to study the Crucifixion. You see, when preachers say that the sin debt was paid in full, to me that meant "in full." Not partially. Jesus didn't die on the cross, thinking, "Ok, I did my part. My death covers just eternal life. Now, you all are on your own until you die." Without referencing a dictionary or thesaurus, I can confidently say that "in full" means "there's nothing I can add to it. It's complete, finished, done, over— The End." You get the picture.

"In full" is then a fundamental concept for us here. The Bible is not a resource that kicks in only after we die. It is for today. It is a guidebook. Everything that sin ushered in, Jesus' blood changed, right?

I believe part of the problem we have with food is that, for many, it has become a strict religion. Food is legalistic. It is based on rules. The focus tends to be on what you are doing wrong and all the food items you need to get out of your diet. We have bought into the belief that it's best to follow the rules because, without them, most people wouldn't know how to feed themselves correctly.

Further, there is also an emerging way of thinking that because food is such a complicated topic, only select people can understand it. Michael Pollan, a food expert and author, has coined this way of thinking as "nutritionism." He says it is "the ideology that food is foremost about nutrition and nutrition is so complex that only experts and industry can supply it." So, where does that leave those who are not experts or industry people?

I like what Mark Batterson says about Jesus in his book *In a Pit with a Lion on a Snowy Day*. If you study the teachings of Christ, you'll realize that learning wasn't His primary goal. His primary goal was unlearning. He was reverse engineering religious minds. And those can be the most difficult minds to change. That is why two phrases are repeated in the Sermon on the Mount. 'You have heard that it was said...' 'But I tell you...'" For a lifetime, we have learned from authorities what we should and should not be eating. That's the "you have heard that it was said" part. Sadly, most of us don't know the "But I tell you..." part. We all believe what the food authorities tell us. And why wouldn't we? They are the experts. But what does God tell you? We believe that food is the primary factor in our health status. We believe that food will make you sick if you get it wrong, and it will heal you if you get it right. Those are big "ifs." How can we reconcile what the experts tell us, for example, in the approximately 120-page 2015–2020 Dietary Guidelines with what Jesus says, "Eat freely." Could it be that simple? Could He be replacing a mistaken or misplaced belief with just one simple statement? That would be Jesus' way. It seems that we have some learning and unlearning yet to do.

What does our Biblical history teach us? What can it

protect us from today? In Hosea 4:6, we read, "My people are destroyed for lack of knowledge." Based on the complexity of food and nutrition today, it would be logical to assume the knowledge we need is about vitamins and minerals, food combining, calorie counting, and macronutrients. But I believe He is referring to the understanding of the full all-encompassing application of the finished work of the cross.

The Christian life should look different if for no other reason than the cross. If we were bought with a price and given Jesus who came that we may have abundant life, shouldn't there be advantages or something that distinguishes our lives from non-believers? But Christians are sick, and they worry about food. They have a dysfunctional relationship with food. Christians suffer from the same confusion and misinformation. Maybe it's because we don't know what the Bible says about food. Interestingly, the answer is simple: it's Jesus.

We, as a culture, have become so food-focused that we are distracted from being cross-focused. If we are cross-focused, then we will be Jesus-focused. Every responsibility we have attributed to food has already been addressed by Jesus, such as healing, reward, pleasure, sickness, comfort, protection, and worry.

Jesus removed the curse from the ground and took away every sickness and disease; He used food to fellowship with His disciples and to remember the cross; He is the Bread of Life. We have divine healing because of the cross, and we can remember this when we take communion. He reinstated for us a relationship with the God who created our food by merely speaking it into existence. He created food before He created man. So logically, He designed our bodies to use the food. We have the promise in Isaiah 54:17, "No weapon formed against you prospers." And He tells us in John 17:14-16 that as Christians, we are in this world, but we are "not of the world." I believe our relationship with food can and should look different.

In Leviticus 2:11, the Bible states, "No grain offering which you bring to the Lord shall be made with leaven." Jesus is our grain offering. He paid it all. He paid for everything. Yet, we live as if we must add to it. The "leaven" referenced here is talking about wrong teachings. Now similarly, this is how Eve got into trouble. She added more to what God said. Remember, Eve told the serpent that they couldn't touch the fruit, adding to God's instruction to simply not eat it. She made it more complicated than it was supposed to be.

We must know what the Bible says about a topic we must consume for survival. Daily, we must make decisions regarding how best to nourish ourselves. What to eat? When to eat? How much to eat? How much to spend? All those questions matter to God because they matter to you. If He cares enough to know how many hairs are on your head (Luke 12:7), then how you nourish yourself is important as well. Remember, He wants you to talk to Him. He wants you to seek Him. He wants to serve you (Matthew 20:28). What you believe about Jesus and the cross truly matters. If you only think that the cross is about getting to Heaven, then you are missing a critical part of His finished work. It cannot be emphasized enough how much food matters to Him.

If your relationship with God is distant, or if you don't fully understand the depth or the benefits, then your relationship with food is likely to be dysfunctional. Remember, with the Lord; there is freedom. He came to set the captive free. He told Adam to eat freely. When Jesus died on the cross, He removed the need for our self-effort. The Ten Commandments were no longer the law of the land. You see, Mount Sinai was about man's ability; man's efforts to keep the rules. In man's imperfection, there was no way he could do it. When Jesus died on the cross, it then became about what Jesus did, His perfection, and who we are in Christ. Who we are has nothing to do with our ability. Daily, we still work hard at eating right. We always abide by a list of self-designed food commandments. Eat three times a day. Don't eat carbohydrates. Eat kale. Just like the Ten Commandments were impossible to keep religiously, food rules and laws are the same. Our God is about freedom.

We have inextricably linked food to health. The Bible doesn't teach this. It does, however, show that health comes from the Word of God (Proverbs 4:22) and the cross. Jesus never asked a person what they ate before He healed them. He never prescribed kale. The consistent factor was Jesus's presence or involvement. It was the spiritual closeness, not the physical proximity. Those who sought Jesus believed He was willing. Some healings were done remotely. Some were done in His presence. Each one was unique. However, the one consistent factor was the relationship between the person asking for healing and the Healer. They knew He could and was willing to do for them what no one else could do. For each person who approached Him for healing, there were greater numbers of people that didn't and missed out for themselves or a loved one. Today, the cross provides us with daily access to the Healer; to the One who took away all sickness and diseases. Your healing has already been purchased, and it wasn't through food.

Now, I have referred to the difference between food and food-like substances. For our purposes in this book, when I refer to food, I am not talking about products made in a lab. These are considered processed foods. With the help of the food industry, the lines between real food and not-so-real food have become blurred. According to Julie Beck in the Atlantic, "More than half of what Americans eat is ultra-processed." Dr. Hyman in the *Food Fix* book tells us "that for every 10% of your diet that is ultra-processed, your risk of death increases by 14%." And "the Standard American Diet is around 60% ultra-processed."[1] The food industry has figured out the more they can process food, the more money they will make from it. Can scientists make edible items that function in the body the same as the food God made? We all know the answer to this question. I am reminded of a joke I heard about a scientist and God. The scientist proudly challenges God to a contest to see who can make a better human being. God happily accepts the challenge. Excited and confident, the scientist goes first. He bends down, picking up dirt, getting ready to fashion his human being. Seeing this, God politely interrupts the process and tells the scientist, "No, no ... you go make your own dirt."

While this is a joke about creating a human, there is an

important point here regarding food. Food made in a lab is not food by the Biblical definition. Contrary to the chemical and lab processing variety, there is something powerful about food that was made by the sound of God's voice. And that food is still being produced today because of the seeds that originated in the Garden. In Genesis 1:11 God said let the earth produce "seed-bearing plants." Due to a host of factors outside the consumer's direct control, our seed variety is diminishing. Dr. Hyman reports, "Between 1903 and 1983, we lost an astonishing 93% of our unique seed varieties. For example, in 1903, there were nearly 500 varieties of lettuce commonly grown; by 1983, that number was down to 36. And that is just one type of crop." The doctor continues to report, "Now, 68% of the remaining seed varieties are in the hands of just three companies globally ... creating farmer dependence on Big Agribusiness ... and destroying seed-saving knowledge amongst generations."

If our food supply is primarily ultra-processed and non-processed foods contain less nutrition than decades ago, while the seed variety is rapidly diminishing and in the hands of just three Agribusiness companies, how are we to adequately feed ourselves? We are supposed to avoid genetically modified foods, but that's the majority of seeds available. It seems we should just be thankful for whatever we can get and should only be prepared to deal with whatever health issues develop as a result. With so many factors outside of our ability to control them, how can we stand a fighting chance to stay healthy and to eat right? Those who are making decisions about our food sources and food quality are much bigger and more powerful than we are. It all feels hopeless.

As a Christian, your Father in Heaven created the food. Let me say the same thing differently. You are a child of the Food Creator. You have an advantage. You have the privilege. You can talk to Him about your food. He knows everything there is to know about food, and He wants to share the information with you. He tells us, "You have not because you ask not" (James 4:2).

James 1:17 tells us, "Whatever is good and perfect is a gift coming down to us from God our Father." In Genesis 1:31, the Bible tells us that, after creating food, God said it was "good." The food was good for Adam. It is still good for us.

Again, I must wonder, if Jesus did all of this on the cross, then why are Christians just as sick as non-Christians? Why is the church an ill place? It seems there's something we don't know or something we are not utilizing. I believe it is a greater understanding and dependence on our relationship with Jesus.

CHAPTER 4

WHY THE EIGHT GIFTS?

Consistent with God's loving nature, and knowing how important food is to our bodies, the Lord provided us with eight gifts to help us relate with and benefit from the original gift He prepared for Adam in the Garden. You see, when God directs you to do something, such as "eat freely," He equips you with the ability and the means to do it. Now, don't get me wrong. He is not expecting you to rely on self-effort to complete His directive. Instead, He partners with you by providing you with the tools to be successful. Isn't that what we all want when it comes to food? We want success in our health quest. Progress in our weight loss. Success in our physical goals. The lack of success is what leads to frustration and resignation. Even from childhood, we learned the lesson that if you misuse something, you forfeit the privilege of using it. Often, because of the misuse, something can become damaged, or someone can even get hurt.

God gave us the gift of food, and we have misused it. We have listened to other opinions and recommendations on how to eat. As a result, sadly, people are getting hurt. In the Garden, there were two trees mentioned: The Tree of Life and the Tree of the Knowledge of Good and Evil. Adam and Eve were forbidden to eat from the latter. It wasn't because the fruit was poisonous or tasted terrible. I believe it was because God didn't want us saddled with the burden of unnecessary knowledge that leads to self-effort. Especially regarding food, more knowledge is not always a good thing. The more we know, the more confused we can become, and the more exasperated we can be testing out the information. As I have said before, we know more details about food today than years ago, but we are in a more significant health crisis. Now, I am not saying that curiosity or wanting to know more about food is a bad thing. I have been interested in and have been studying food for years. It's not that the knowledge is terrible. The problem occurs when the knowledge takes precedence over the truth. Simply, sometimes knowledge and truth don't align. Frequently, I began to see the conflict between what I was studying and what I was reading in the Bible. For me, the full understanding of food had to include what the Bible said.

In August 1982, a book was published entitled *Og Mandino's University of Success* by Og Mandino. It was a compilation of advice from successful men and women, or in Og's words, "the fifty brilliant minds" to produce "the ultimate success book." On the topic of knowledge, in 1969, Cavett Robert writes, "Knowledge is accumulating so fast and methods of doing things improving so rapidly that a person today must run to stand still. Up to 1900, it was said that the accumulation of knowledge doubled every century. At the end of World War II, knowledge doubled every twenty-five years. Today all the research centers tell us that the volume of knowledge in existence doubles every five years. Where does that leave the person today who thinks he can stand still and survive?" That question was asked 50 years ago. Today we have the internet, which exponentially increases our exposure to knowledge. Mr. Robert goes on to say, "What was not only right but even plausible yesterday, is questionable today and might even be wrong tomorrow." Knowledge is vast, but it is ever-changing. We must be careful.

Then we have the Tree of Life. This tree was not off-limits. God wanted Adam and Eve to feed on it. Its fruit was life and all things related to life. The same instructions apply to us today. We read in Proverbs 4:20-22, "My son, attend to my words; incline thy ear unto my sayings. Let them not depart from thy eyes; keep them amid thy heart. For they are life unto those that find them, and health to all their flesh." Isn't this what we are after? It's not about more knowledge of what is good or bad. It's about focusing on the source of life, which is God's Word. Amid all the opinions and studies about food, we should consider what the Bible says about it.

There is such great physical and spiritual benefit to the food we eat that God doesn't want us overwhelmed or frustrated by its complexity. The food's complexity is in the Lord's hands. He knows exactly what that food contains and in the proper ratios. Let's take any herb, for example. This plant can consist of hundreds or thousands of naturally occurring chemicals. According to research, some of these chemicals have synergistic effects on the other chemicals, increasing their activity. At the same time, other present chemicals modify the results of other chemicals thereby reducing undesirable side effects. This demonstrates that we have no control over food's complexity. The delicate balance of plant constituents is not up to us. Scientists have become frustrated by the fact that, even though they may be able to isolate an active ingredient in a specific food item such as an herb, they can't reproduce its effectiveness on its own. In fact, by itself, that specific isolated chemical can cause harm without the other mitigating synergistic components. There is a delicate balance. The effectiveness and the safety of that food require the other ingredients found within that same food source. This requirement has God's creative fingerprints all over it. While there is nothing wrong with science, it has limitations. It will never fully be able to analyze food at the God-level. However, I do believe that God gives man the ability to analyze and to formulate chemicals that provide a medicinal benefit, but man will always have limits. So, while food is complicated to us it is no problem for the Creator. Remember, He created it with just a word.

God doesn't want us worried about the food complexity or chasing knowledge to try to understand something that is beyond our ability to know. We can and have learned a lot about food composition and benefits, but we still don't have all the answers. The Lord doesn't want us to struggle. As a result, He has provided us a simple solution. It's not about a mathematical caloric formula or even the latest diet trend. It's knowing who we are because of Jesus and functioning fully in the additional gifts purchased at the cross.

Despite Adam's disobedience, God did not leave man to find his way back to God on his own. Nor did God step back frustrated with man's disobedience and passive-aggressively say, "figure it out yourself." Quite the contrary. He provided for us eight gifts that will help us in our relationship to food. Our present dysfunctional relationship with food breaks God's heart. According to Dr. Mark Hyman, "6 in 10 adults in the U. S. have a chronic disease, 4 in 10 have two or more. Eleven million people die each year from eating bad food, and it's preventable. The food we eat is the number one cause of death in the world. Mental health is one of the biggest crises in America today, and a lot of the problem is driven by food." Dr. Hyman's statistics bear repeating: "60% of our calories come from ultra-processed foods like flour, sugar, wheat, corn and soybean oil. The people who eat the most of these are the sickest. For every 10% of the diet that's ultra-processed food, your risk of death goes up by 14%." In their quest to sell convenience, the food industry repeatedly reinforces the idea that cooking is inconvenient, expensive, and takes up too much of your precious time. There is a lot of knowledge accumulating among the food industry, scientists, marketers, and physicians. The problem is not a lack of knowledge. The dysfunctional relationship is entirely unnecessary. Rest assured; God sees the struggle. He knows food matters to us. He designed us to need it. Thankfully, in Joshua 1:8, He has promised to give us "good success."

Now, ironically, these are gifts that we learned in church,

but only regarding spiritual things. Because of the cross, these eight gifts are already ours. We don't have to earn them or buy them. As Christians, we already have them. They are guaranteed for success. The problem is that in the church, you typically don't hear preachers talk about it, especially in the context of food. Yet, most of the congregation is struggling somehow with food. These gifts are advantages that the Christian has only because of the cross. They are fail-proof tools we can use to have a healthy relationship with food.

But as we have seen so far, there are two distinct sides to the food coin. There is a spiritual and a physical consequence or reaction to everything. The same goes for food. Remember, Adam and Eve physically ate the fruit ushering in a spiritual and physical death and separation from God.

After all the years of attending church and studying the Bible, I never really thought about the topic of food. I learned the Bible is a living, breathing document that is just as relevant and applicable today as it was back in Biblical times. So, when I was studying for my Master's, individual spiritual tenants about food would come to mind. For example, considering the different diets and learning the rules of each, I would recall that the Bible says, "eat freely." I just couldn't ignore or shake the contradiction. I hear people often talking about the details of the specific diet they are on at that moment. Given the opportunity to vent, they will inevitably remark about how tired they are of being hungry. The scenario typically plays out the same way. They have a weak moment, eat whatever they want, then cope with the guilt and shame of being a self-described failure. Even despite

Adam's sin, the Lord would never call him a failure. He can't see us that way. Instead, the Lord sees us for who we are in Him. We can do all things. We are more than conquerors. Yet, somehow, in the context of food, we don't speak the same language as the Lord. We don't see ourselves as victorious or triumphant.

In the Old Testament, because the Israelites were so convinced that they could keep all the laws, they asked for the Ten Commandments. In Exodus 19:7-8, we read, "So Moses went back and summoned the elders of the people and set before them all the words the Lord had commanded him to speak. The people all responded together 'We will do everything the Lord has said.'" This is a crucial point to dissect here. Anytime someone is given a list of rules, even in a diet, there is an initial belief that, in and of yourself, you will be able to follow them to the letter. You believe in your capability, and you want the positive results. At the onset, typically a Monday, or on the first of January, everyone starts like gangbusters. You follow the rules to the letter, until lunchtime, inconvenience, hunger, boredom, or the reluctant admittance of failure occurs.

God didn't design us to navigate life without complete dependence on Him. When we go it alone, we are destined to fail. That's just how it is. He created man for fellowship. Every detail of your life that matters to you matters to Him because He loves you more than you can imagine. Strangely, there is security in rules. But when they are too rigid or unrealistic, it showcases our limitations and inability to be perfect. When we rely on self-effort or our knowledge of what we think is right or wrong, we will ultimately fail. The Ten Commandments show us this. As soon as one of the Israelites took something that belonged to another person, no matter how small the item, they broke the Commandment "Thou Shall Not Steal." The very moment that one of the Israelites disrespected a parent, they broke the Commandment "Thou Shall Honor Thy Father and Thy Mother." There were deadly consequences of not keeping every one of the Ten Commandments. If you broke one Commandment, you broke them all. Truthfully, what the Ten Commandments served to do was showcase man's inability to be perfect in his self-effort.

It seems odd, but we are drawn to rules with the optimistic belief or hope that "I can do it this time." Maybe it's to prove something to ourselves or other people. There's nothing wrong with that belief in ourselves. But that's just the point; it's a belief in yourself.

One of the recent shifts in thinking about weight loss, which is the sole reason people begin diets, is that diets typically don't work. Over the years, there have been numerous diets that have come and gone. It's a good bet the diets of today will suffer the same fate and will rarely be heard of in years to come. So now the mantra is "a lifestyle change." The Lord doesn't want us to live by rules. If He did, He would have never sent Jesus. There are several references to the "stone" tablets of the Ten Commandments. In the Bible, the stone represents the law. The law is the antithesis to grace.

Let us take, for example, the simple rule of eating three times a day. Research shows that the food industry is responsible for introducing that little nugget into our daily things-to-do. Now I am not here to dispute whether that is sound advice or not. Suffice it to say; I couldn't find that in the Bible anywhere. In certain circles, you hear experts saying that you must eat six times a day. So, which one is it? Which rule do you follow?

Another example is the Nutritional Guidelines that are written and dispensed by the government to tell people what they should and should not eat. They inform you how much and what type of fat you should consume, how many carbohydrates, how much water to drink, and even more detail than you'll probably ever want to know. According to ChooseMyPlate.com, "The 2015–2020 Dietary Guidelines for Americans emphasize the importance of creating a healthy eating pattern to maintain health and reduce the risk of disease. Everything we eat and drink — the food and beverage choices we make day to day and over our lifetime — matters." I can agree with that. A final example of self-imposed rules is "Breakfast is the most important meal of the day." Once this circulated through mainstream, people were waking up and forcing food down their throats even if they weren't hungry. While this is not phrased as a dogmatic "You will eat breakfast" to a person who is trying to make healthy choices, this is more than a nudge in that direction. Just so you know, research shows that John Kellogg, MD., was responsible for that advice. He had formulated a recipe for breakfast cereals that his brother Will took to market. Was there a conflict of interest? Was the motivation to sell it to the masses strictly the health of the consumer? If so, that would be

"GRRREAT," but according to The Food That Built America film, the motivation was strictly competition with Post cereal and profit.

Doctors, nutritionists, and other health professionals base their advice on the government's Dietary Guidelines. Doctors, with very few hours of nutrition study in medical school, tell their patients what to eat. I've even personally overheard doctors give patients dietary advice based on how they themselves eat. If a vegetarian diet works for them, they believe everyone should eat that way too! In one case, I heard a doctor tell a patient to stop eating anything with eyes or feet. This doctor was recovering from leukemia and was advising all his patients to eat the way he does. He never checked to see if the patient would do well on a vegetarian diet or not.

The Dietary Guidelines influence National School Lunch Programs and the Nutritional Program for Women, Infants, and Children (WIC). These Guidelines have a far-reaching impact. So, you would expect them to be correct. According to nutritioncoalition.us, the "Guidelines are undoubtedly the single most influential lever on our food supply as well as our ideas about what constitutes a healthy diet." But sadly, as time has passed, information is continuing to come to light that the Guidelines were motivated more by profit for some rather than the health of the American people. Philip Handler, President of the National Academy of Sciences from 1969–1981, is quoted as saying, "What right has the federal government to propose that the American people conduct a vast nutritional experiment with themselves as subjects, on the strength of so little evidence?"

Remember my point that chasing knowledge can sometimes lead to people getting hurt? The Dietary Guidelines launched in 1980. Coincidentally, that year marked the rise in the percentage of the U.S. overweight and obesity statistics. The numbers have yet to decline.

People are, to some extent, trying to adhere to these Guidelines. They have become indoctrinated into our way of thinking. However, there is widespread criticism about the lack of scientific evidence.

The first Guidelines launched in 1980, based on a 1977 report by the Senate Select Committee on Nutrition called Dietary Goals for Americans. The Senate report recommended that Americans should consume less fat (particularly saturated fat), less dietary cholesterol, and more grains, fruits, and vegetables. This recommendation is the same advice that we are given today.

This Senate report that started it all, later came under scrutiny, as it was written by a single staffer who favored vegetarianism. According to Science Magazine (2001), "It was Senator George McGovern's bipartisan, non-legislative Select Committee on Nutrition and Human Needs — and, to be precise, a handful of McGovern's staff members — that almost single-handedly changed nutritional policy in this country and initiated the process of turning the dietary fat hypothesis into dogma."

Nina Teicholz, the author of *The Big Fat Surprise*, writes: "It's hard to overstate what a radical departure from the government's stand on nutrition the Dietary Guidelines for Americans represented when it first came out in 1980. Since 1956, the USDA had been advising people to seek out nutritious foods by eating a 'well-balanced' diet of the basic food groups first five of them, then seven, then four. The four food groups were milk, meat, fruits & vegetables, and cereals & grains. Americans had been encouraged to eat some foods from each group every day. The USDA has always suffered from a conflict of interest, since it's entire mission is to promote American food commodities, and the agency has long been heavily influenced by those very industries."

So, the advice we have been given has been biasedly motivated. No wonder people don't know what to eat or who to trust for that matter.

As wanna-be rule followers, it's hard to know what to eat. You genuinely try, then you don't get the results you want. Then, just like in the Land of Oz, when you peek behind the nutritional curtain, you realize that your health is not the primary focus of many of those pulling the levers and telling you what you should and shouldn't eat. There is a lot of political and financial peddling going on while you're standing in the middle of the grocery store trying to decide if "heart-healthy" really means heart healthy. Who can you trust with your food anymore? I'll tell you, the Creator of the food Himself. He is not swayed by profit or greed. There is no bias. He's not trying to manufacture cheap food or create a chemical cocktail that tastes like cheese. Just for kicks and giggles, next time you are opening the cheese wrapper to put that yellow slice on your sandwich, take a look at the back of the packaging to see if it says something similar to "imitation cheese product." Yum, yum. By the way, in 2013, this imitation cheese product was labeled a health food for kids.[1]

While the topic of food has become so complicated, considering the complexity, the bias, the wrong advice, and the ever-changing recommendations, the solution seems simple yet strangely not-so-obvious: nourishing our bodies with food created by a God who has no ulterior motive. He is not out to become CEO of a mega food company, and He is not interested in chemically engineering the genetic DNA of food. He did it right the first time and saw no need to improve upon it. He wants to nourish you. He wants to bless you. He wants you to enjoy what you eat. He wants you to include Him. He made that way possible. Sadly, for most Christians, we just didn't realize it was there all this time. Over the years, we have put our faith in everything else, including ourselves, when it comes to food. While the trust has been misplaced, there's a way to get back to the way it is supposed to be.

He knows you personally. He knows how your body works uniquely. He knows what your body needs at this very moment. Talk to Him. Listen to Him. Let Him guide you to understand what your body needs. Stand on His promises for protection and health. Jesus is the answer to all the responsibilities we have assigned to food. In Psalm 32:8, He promises, "I will instruct you and teach you in the way you should go." It's as easy as a daily walk with Him.

Man's involvement with food has caused physical and spiritual confusion and damage. The more damage is done, the more we attribute the cause of our declining health to what we eat. Conversely, we look to food to fix it. There is something special about the food that God created. Remember, He spoke it into existence. I believe that it still hears His voice. It recognizes His words even when we are the ones speaking it. Food knows God's language. It knows its Creator. For example, when Jesus turned water into wine, where did the grapes come from? The grapes fast-tracked the fermenting process to become the best wine at the wedding.

Interestingly, a miracle involving food was the first miracle Jesus performed. I believe it is because He knows how important food is to us and to demonstrate that He is still in control of it. But He lets man be part of it. In John 2:1-11, we read the story of the wedding in Galilee attended by Jesus and His mother. When she brought the socially devastating news to Jesus that "They have no more wine," he could have snapped His fingers and solved the problem. Instead, Jesus' mother instructed the servants to do what is relevant for us today: "Do whatever He tells you." You see, they could have devised their plan to fix this problem. They could have gone to the store to buy more. They could have had close friends go home and retrieve whatever wine stash they had. But instead, Jesus's way produced a better result. He has control over the grapes, over time, and over your food, too. Just "do whatever He tells you." He has told us to "Eat freely."

God created food for pleasure. Yet, you rarely hear of anyone enjoying their food. And when you do, it is typically accompanied by some level of guilt and the rhetorical questions, "Why did I do that?" or "Why did I eat so much?" In fact, I have read on social media the statement that "Food never tastes as good as skinny feels." What a statement! We have learned that we are not supposed to enjoy food. Instead, the satisfaction is found in our long-term adherence to craving denials and self-sacrifice. We tell ourselves, "It will all be worth it when I lose the last 5 pounds!" We then revert to the previous way of eating, which resulted in the weight issue. It's the dysfunctional love-hate relationship.

The more that government and man have gotten involved in the food, the more advice we take from "authorities," and the more we apply what those trusted authorities recommend, the sicker we are becoming. Just like Eve, we turned the reigns over to another. We aren't quite sure what the Bible says about food, so we accept what others tell us. But truthfully, it's not an either-or-situation. We can, just like Eve, blend Biblical information with the worldly authority resulting in one big, giant mess. Just a random thought, has anyone ever wondered why Eve was standing next to the forbidden tree if she thought she wasn't supposed to touch it? What was so enticing?

Was she looking at the fruit when the serpent saw her? Did she position herself in a vulnerable place, opening the door for the serpent? No matter what led up to their interaction, the consequences for Eve were severe. Our effects today are critical as well. People are sick, and they are dying. The Bible says, "My people will be destroyed for lack of knowledge." I believe this means the right knowledge. It's time to change that.

While we will be discussing eight gifts to help us develop a healthy relationship with food, God, in His love and mercy, doesn't require us to be proficient at using all of them at once. Just learning to implement one can and will make a difference. Like with any project, the more tools you become adept at using, the easier the task, and the better the results. And these gifts are not mutually exclusive. They enhance each other beautifully. There's no pressure to get it right. Remember, in this regard, your success has nothing to do with your efforts. It's learning to rest in the finished work of the cross and to operate in the gifts you have as a Christian.

He wants us to be successful in all that we do. He wants us healthy and fit for His purpose. He has things for us to accomplish. If we don't feel well or don't have the energy or are preoccupied or consumed with thoughts of food and self-image, then we are less than effective. We are to stand in the victory of the cross and take back the gift of food. He has made a way and provided us with the tools to do it. Better yet, He promises that we will be successful; that He will give us success. Let's get started!

CHAPTER 5

GRACE

In Genesis chapter 6, we read of how wicked mankind had become since the advent of sin. In verse 5, "The Lord saw how great the wickedness of the human race had become on the earth ... The Lord regretted that he had made human beings ... and his heart was deeply troubled." In verse 7, we read of the Lord's plans." I will wipe from the face of the earth the human race I have created ... for I regret that I have made them." In verse 8, we read, "Noah found grace in the eyes of the Lord." The use of the word "grace" in this verse is the first mention of grace in the Bible. So, the context of its use is worth unpacking. Notice that grace coincided with the Lord's worst feelings toward man. He was troubled and regretted creating human beings, but "Noah found grace."

For a broader understanding, the word "grace" is also interpreted as "favor" in other Biblical translations. Grace is an advantage. Simply defined, it is His kindness when we don't deserve it. We get a benefit we didn't work for or earn. It is an important concept for Christians to understand, especially since "grace" is one of the most widely used words in the Bible.

Grace is one of those spiritual concepts that apply to a person's salvation. Because of God's undeserved favor, you won't spend eternity in hell after you die. In Ephesians 2:8-9, we read, "For by grace are ye saved through faith; and that not of yourselves: it is the gift of God. Not of works, lest any man should boast." God's grace required Jesus's death on the cross so that we could spend eternity with Him. It also has an application for us in our daily living. And food plays a big part in that.

There is a widely held belief that food heals the body. Think about it. If God designed our bodies to function on His creation, then when we eat it, there's a prescribed and God-designed benefit. When a person becomes sick, certain foods are quickly prescribed, and others are restricted. For example, when a friend of mine was diagnosed with cancer, her physician, as part of her treatment, began radically changing her diet. She was told to avoid red meat and to start eating more vegetables. She was also instructed not to eat black pepper. The doctor believed it formed an impenetrable coating around the tumors preventing the body from being able to attack it.

Typically, people battling cancer are told to eat an alkaline diet and drink alkaline water. While there may be some truth or scientific reasoning behind this dietary advice, from the Biblical standpoint, no food was ever prescribed for a sick person. In fact, in Mark 5:21-43, we read the story of Jesus healing the little girl. Only after the healing does he instruct her family to give her something to eat. Jesus didn't recommend the specific food that scientists had recently determined to have the exact healing properties this little girl needed. He didn't even ask what she had been eating before getting sick. For Jesus, it didn't matter.

When someone has been eating unhealthy food and then becomes sick, we tend to think that they brought it on themselves. Grace isn't a green light to eat junk and to treat your body unhealthily. But when you are following God's instruction to eat freely of the food He has created, He covers you with His grace. Under His undeserved favor, your body will benefit beyond what the food can do. The little girl didn't get better because of food. She got better because of Jesus.

Hippocrates said, "Let thy food be they medicine, and thy medicine be thy food." Our culture has reached a point where what you eat is blamed or credited for every illness and every recovery. Even then, it is still a guessing game. A person can eat a natural diet and exercise religiously yet die young. How do you know when you've gotten it right? If the focus is on your food alone, you'll never know for sure. This difficulty has contributed to our food-focused obsession, sadly, to the exclusion of the Food Creator.

Interestingly, the first mention of grace in the Bible concerns Noah and the Flood. The name "Noah" means "rest." Therefore, Genesis 6:8 could potentially read, "Rest found grace in the eyes of the Lord." When it comes to food, how many people do you know who are at rest? How many do you know who are frequently worried about their health and what they eat? What God is telling us here is that when we come to the place of rest, when we stop struggling and trying to rely on ourselves to eat right or to lose the weight, God's grace or favor is more than enough. He wants us to talk to and involve Him. He wants us to include Him, and most importantly, to trust Him. Remember, grace is God's kindness that we don't deserve. The emphasis is kindness. It's a benefit we didn't work for.

Often the terms grace and mercy are used interchangeably. But their meanings are vastly different. Grace is about getting something positive we didn't deserve. Mercy is not experiencing the punishment or the negative consequence we should have. The differences are subtle but significant. Because of the cross, every area of the Christian's life is covered in grace. And we are shielded from sin's consequences by mercy. Do Christians know that? Do we operate in His grace and favor?

Here's a practical example of the difference between grace and mercy. Because of Adam's sin, we are separated from God and will spend eternity in hell. Grace supplies us with the relationship with God and eternity with Him in Heaven. Neither of which we deserve. Mercy keeps us from living eternity in hell. So, grace gives us heaven; mercy keeps us from hell. It's subtle. But like I said earlier, it's significant.

On our own, we get tired of focusing on food. We are bombarded with messages, advertisements, and social media posts, keeping us committed to our effort to eat right and stay healthy. The repetitive cycle of trying new diets only to find that it is not sustainable long term, resulting in feelings of guilt, shame, and failure when you quit, are landmarks on the all too familiar, well-trodden trip around that same mountain. This path is crowded with people believing this time will be different. But, demonstrated time and again, there are limits to how long you can adhere to those rules. But God's grace has no limits. It has no expiration. He gives us new grace every day. Just like when the Israelites were in the Wilderness, God provided manna for them to gather every morning. He promised to care for them. Yet, the only requirement was that they were not to collect the manna and store it for the next day. If they did, it bred worms and began to smell (Exodus 16:13-20). Collecting the food to keep for the next day demonstrated that they were anticipating their needs for tomorrow instead of letting an all-knowing God handle the need when the day came. He didn't want the Israelites worrying about their food. He promised to take care of His chosen people, and He did. He wants you to rest in the knowledge that, as a Christian, you live under the grace purchased by the cross. That grace gives you a decisive advantage activated by resting in Him.

People typically focus on food because of health reasons. Our society today draws a direct correlation between your health and the food you eat. It is imperative that you get it right, and time is of the essence. Under grace, you can rest in knowing that your Heavenly Father knows what you need and will guide you. If He has led you to eat a certain way and to let go of certain food addictions, He will give you the grace to do it. Remember, grace is a benefit you didn't work to get. It has nothing to do with your self-effort. Just like with the Israelites and the manna, self-effort never produces the results He can. No one wants stinky, wormy food! Your health, your energy, your ability to do what He has called you to do matters to Him, and He will equip you with all the grace you need. His grace will even cover for the mistakes you will inevitably make. He's not expecting perfection. You don't have to work for grace. Instead of struggling to lose weight or working hard to eat right, Hebrews 4:11 tells us "Let us, therefore, make every effort to enter that rest." Then the grace will flow.

Let's apply this to a practical example. When we function in God's grace, our health is not as directly correlated to our food choices. Resting in Him, He will guide you on how to eat. The focus is removed from the food and instead shifted to your Heavenly Father. Society tells us if we eat poorly, we are going to get sick, and our food choices will have caused our health issues. But grace teaches something to the contrary. Now, this is not an invitation to eat whatever you want. We know that processed foods are calorically dense, nutritionally void, and laden with human-made chemicals our bodies are not well-equipped to handle. His grace covers our imperfections. We will never have the ideal diet 100% of the time. In truth, no one knows what the perfect diet is. Instead, His food and His grace are all we need.

In Biblical numerology, the number five represents God's grace. It is also a number that symbolizes God's kindness and favor to humankind. As if grace wasn't sufficient enough, in

John 1:16, we read, "From His fullness, we have all received grace upon grace." So, when we need more grace, He's ready and willing to provide it. No matter what, you simply can't exhaust His grace supply.

Based on the sin in the Garden, we deserve to work for our food, struggle with eating, and suffer the inevitable consequences. Along with Adam's disobedience, we inherited Adam's punishment. As Christians, because of the cross, we can instead rely on His grace. I believe that when you have an awareness of His grace in connection with your food and health, you begin to recognize the gift of the food He created for your body. You find ways to incorporate more of His provision into your daily life. Honestly, the lure of convenience and calorically dense, highly palatable food is strong. It's downright addictive. It was designed in the lab by scientists working for the food industry giants specifically for that purpose. The food manufacturers make a lot of money if they addict you to needing more of their food. But even if that is your current situation, God's grace is big enough to cover that too. Rest in Him. Stop struggling to overcome food addiction on your own — partner with Him. When you rest and rely on Him, the results are up to Him. Bring grace into your desire to give up the addiction. You just need to get to your place of rest.

When researching food in Genesis, I referenced the Strongest NIV Exhaustive Concordance for the first four uses of the word "food" in the Garden. In context, they each refer to the fruit or food provided for Adam before the fall. Interestingly, the fifth reference to food is translated "bread."

This reference was made when God was outlining to Adam the consequences he deserved because of his disobedience. This is when Adam found out that, going forward, he would have to work for his food. Now, remember, the number five symbolizes grace. Adam didn't know that, in years to come, Jesus would be known as the Bread of Life. Isn't that amazing? In God's grace, when His heart was at its most broken because He lost fellowship with Adam, He immediately instituted Adam's grace. It was Jesus. It was the Bread. Isn't that exciting?

God wants us to relate to our food with grace. It is essential to understand that the presence of our food is here by His grace. In the Garden, God commanded the ground to produce food. When Adam sinned, the Lord could have told the ground to stop. But He permitted it to continue producing. Imagine where we'd be if the earth were told to stop producing food. We would plant a seed, and 100 years later, that seed would still be sitting there, dormant, and lifeless. We take for granted that the earth produces what we plant. We tend to think that it's what the ground does. It always has. Because of His love for us, in our most sinful state, knowing that He created our bodies to function best on His creation, He allowed the earth to still produce food for us. What does this say about food that is produced in a lab? Or food that the government requires to be outfitted with a label and a list of ingredients? The earth didn't produce it. God didn't make it. A scientist in a lab did. God knew that we needed food. When we eat what was created for us, it is covered with a sprinkling of grace.

The Lord knew the importance of the provision of real food for our bodies, so much so that He made sure to protect it. He cursed the earth, but then shed Jesus's blood on the ground to cancel the curse. In the church, we are taught what a world without grace would be. We would all live eternity in hell. When Christians realize grace also covers activity of daily life, such as the production of the food and how our body uses the food, it sweetens the meaning and understanding of the gift of grace.

When sickness or death entered the world as a result of sin, God didn't create a new batch of food. The DNA of the food He created didn't change. Our DNA changed. We didn't need different foods to address the newly introduced sickness and death. Instead, He sent his Son.

The Lord can multiply the health benefits of what He created. He still has complete control over His creation. He has no obligation to increase the nutritional benefits of what man created. That's not to say that in His loving-kindness, He wouldn't. God knows your situation. Invite Him into your nutritional decisions and choices and watch what He will do just for you.

When I was in private school, we were taught about the concept of grace. While I don't recall the specific grade school year, I do remember the teacher standing in front of the classroom and asking, "What is grace?" Collectively and in unison, my classmates and I would say, "Grace is God's kindness to us when we deserve punishment." I can still remember it after all these years. Something always bothered me about that phrase. To a child hearing this definition, or maybe to anyone believing that God is primed and ready to strike, the emphasis tends to fall on the word "punishment." The punishment always meant "hell." In our context today, it could also mean sickness. We don't hear the kindness part. We expect the punishment part.

I heard a sermon by a pastor talking about how God took care of the Israelites in the Wilderness. The pastor stated that when the Israelites journeyed from Egypt to Mount Sinai, they were under the Abrahamic covenant of grace. They only came under the law when the Ten Commandments were given to them at Mount Sinai. Likewise, when we impose regulations of any kind, it supplants His grace. When we try to follow diet rules, we lapse into self-effort. To be successful, we must abide by them to the strictest letter. Our diet success is based on how well we can do that. The emphasis is on us. For the Christian, God never assigned a diet as we know it today in the Bible. The Old Testament outlines the dietary laws of the Jewish people. There's the Daniel fast. But they are specific for a group of people or a person. And they were God-given. Diets are so commonplace in our culture that it is hard to believe there was ever a time when they didn't exist. My nutrition studies revolved around foods and specific ways of eating, depending upon the goal or the health need. Every generation can name the popular diet at the time. The menus from the 70's look different from the foods of the '80s and '90s. Years ago, people drank something called Tab. People tried the cabbage soup diet. Everyone decided to go low fat or no fat. Then there was Atkins. Now there's Keto. There will be others.

While we are focused on what to eat and what to avoid, the Lord is always concentrated on grace. It's how He operates. In 2 Corinthians 9:8, we read, "And God is able to make all grace abound toward you, that you, always having all sufficiency in all things, may have an abundance for every good work." The more grace you need, the more grace He gives. It's unlimited. And it is there the precise moment you need it. When we are aware of this inexhaustible, abundant supply of grace, we can come to a place of rest. He doesn't want you stressing about your food. If His grace is powerful enough to keep us out of hell, then it is powerful enough to help you fight junk food addictions and sugar cravings. I'm just saying.

We are told in Hebrews 4:16, "Let us then approach God's throne of grace with confidence, so that we may receive mercy and find grace to help us in our time of need." Arguably, the confusion and damage done by food constitutes a time of need. Because this is a Bible verse, we typically assume it only applies to the spiritual aspects of our life. This causes us to miss a powerful and practical application for the "life abundant" that Jesus died to give us (John 10:10). It is predicted that in 35 years, the health care costs in the US will be $95 trillion. That's trillion with a "T." Based on that alone, it doesn't appear that the experts are expecting the problem to get much better. We have picked up momentum in declining health despite strenuous efforts; not much is changing. To me, this constitutes a need.

Food frustrates people. Typically, when people diet, they do so because there is a physical need, whether it be to lose weight or to regain their health. Remember His invitation to come confidently to the throne of grace and let Him give you all the nutritional benefits that you don't deserve concerning food: health, energy, and a changed perspective about food. It will never be because you deserve it. It's because He purchased the gift of grace for you on the cross.

Having the right relationship with food is best defined as eating what is right for you because you feel led to do it. This approach is much different than trying to eat healthily or cut calories because you are "supposed to" do it. There is no grace in believing you must or have to do anything. I am not saying that changing the way you eat is not part of regaining your health or losing weight. But come boldly to the throne and ask for His grace that will guide you to adopt the approach He knows is best for you. Do you have this confidence?

You're not coming on your terms or qualifications. Instead, you're coming on Jesus's. The grace you need is there for you to take and as much as you need. Grace covers your mistakes. Rest in the fact that you don't have to be perfect because Jesus is.

Some critics say that operating under grace gives people a license to sin and get away with it. But with a greater understanding of grace, you don't beat yourself up when you do sin. Even with grace, no one's perfect. I believe the same applies to food. Living under a greater awareness of grace doesn't give you a free ticket to eat whatever you want. Instead, drawing closer to the One Who created your food gives you a greater appreciation for what He designed your body to optimally utilize for fuel. When you have a greater understanding and appreciation of what is yours because of the cross and the benefits of the cross, it changes how you see food.

You come boldly to the throne of grace, where there is more grace than you will ever need for whatever your dietary situation. When you come boldly, it means not being timid. You have a blood-bought right and secure relationship with the Grace-giver. He has promised to give you the grace you need every day without limit. When it comes to food, you don't have to struggle. We struggle when there's too much information to decipher. Approach the throne knowing that the cross entitles you to kindness you don't deserve. That kindness comes in the form of advantages and benefits that you didn't work for. When you rest in the fact that you have what you need, resting in Jesus, it keeps the river of grace flowing directly to you.

The gift of grace is a tool that the Christian can utilize to benefit in all aspects of their life, both spiritual and physical. The more you learn to rest in His grace, the more He makes available. Grace provides the freedom to let go of the limited self-effort that results in frustration and exhaustion. It provides us with all the benefits we didn't earn. Even on our best day, we could never earn what grace can give us. Just rest — accept His invitation to come to His throne of grace — the place that will transform your relationship to food. Find rest and eat freely.

CHAPTER 6

RIGHTEOUSNESS

When someone comments, "That person acts entitled," it's never intended as a compliment. Even if it's preceded or followed by the mark of a potential southern criticism "Bless their heart ..." the message is still the same. Today, the older generations accuse the millennial generation and younger of this quite often. Behavior associated with entitlement is very unflattering and, frankly, off-putting. The entitled person believes they are owed something just because they exist. Brian Buffini, a real estate mogul, personal growth personality, and host of the Brian Buffini podcast, talks about the entitled character in the realm of business. Entitled people have a sense that they don't need to start at the bottom of the ladder, so to speak. Typically, they don't want to answer to authority either. Sadly, you don't have to be a millennial to act entitled. Buffini says that a great way to know whether you suffer from entitlement is if you complain. If you complain about something, it is because you feel entitled to a different outcome or response.

While the accusation of entitlement is not a flattering description, as Christians, we are supposed to live entitled. We are to boldly declare 2 Corinthians 5:21 that I am the righteousness of God in Christ Jesus. When we realize our righteousness and all that status entitles us to, it's a game-changer.

In Proverbs 12:28, we read, "In the way of the righteousness is life, and in its pathway, there is no death."

Jesus is our righteousness. Because of Him, we are entitled. On our own, we deserve a crushing sin debt that we can never repay. So being righteously entitled, our lives should look substantially different from those who don't know Jesus. In Exodus 8:23, we read of the Israelites living in the land of Egypt. The Israelites were God's chosen people. When God sent plagues over Egypt to get Pharaoh's attention to free the Israelites from slavery, God declared, "I will make a difference between My people and your people." It's the same today.

As Christians, we are God's people. We are children of the Most High God. He wants us to stand out. He wants us to look and act entitled. He wants there to be a visible difference in the way His children's lives look compared to others. Righteousness is what sets you apart.

The more you understand your righteousness or your right standing with God, the more comfortable you will be basking in a personal relationship with Him. You will expect the promises in His Word to be your promises. You are entitled to those outcomes. 2 Corinthians 1:20 tells us, "For no matter how many promises God has made, they are 'Yes' in Christ. And so, through him, the 'Amen' is spoken by us to the glory of God." In other words, we can stand on every promise and will say "Amen" to the outcome. So, say it loud and proud, "I am entitled to all of His promises because I am the righteousness of God in Christ Jesus!" Now your acting entitled, bless your heart! (Don't worry, it's used here as a genuine southern compliment.)

In Proverbs 11:30, "The fruit of the righteous is a tree of life." Remember the Tree of Life is the other tree named in the Garden. The fruit of this tree is life. Jesus came that we may have life abundant. In John 10:10, we read, "I have come that they might have life and that they may have it more abundantly." Think about that for a moment.

You are entitled to an abundant life. Part of daily life is eating. God wants you to enjoy the experience abundantly. To have life abundant, you can't be sick or have low energy. He wants you abundantly healthy, abundantly nourished, and abundantly energetic.

Romans 5:17 captures the connection between the Garden and the Crucifixion for which this book is based. "For if by the one man's offense death reigned through the one much more those who receive abundance of grace and the gift of righteousness will reign in life through the One, Jesus Christ." We tend to think that references to life mean merely continuing to breathe or the drudgeries of every day, such as work, finances, responsibilities, and opportunities. But food is also a part of our daily life. Without it, we won't have life or, at least for a short period, not a quality one.

So, if we are righteous, then we should behave entitled. Entitled not because of who or what you are, but because of what He's done. As a Christian, you can't take off the robe of righteousness, but you can fail to operate in its power. You can behave contrary to someone wearing the robe of righteousness. Meaning, even if you are wearing the robe, that you can live the way the rest of the world does. Mark Twain said it best when he quipped, "Clothing makes the man." Any fashion designer knows that when you put on an attractive outfit, you stand taller. You feel more confident. What you wear affects how you think about yourself and influences the decisions you make. When you are dressed right, you are proud to present yourself to others. You know you look good. And you know that people see you looking good.

When my grandmother would come to stay with us for a week, my husband liked to tease her. Often, this would occur while she would be getting ready for us to take her out somewhere. She'd be in her bathroom, fixing her hair in the mirror. My husband would enter the bathroom and position himself beside her. He'd then pretend to be startled and holler "Oh no, Mema! It happened again!" Forgetting that he did the same thing during her last visit, she would always become alarmed and would then respond, "What! What happened?" He would mischievously grin and answer, "I just got better looking." Realizing she fell for it again; she would laugh and slap at his back as he walked out of the bathroom. God wants us to operate in that same confidence every day because we are wearing the robe of righteousness. And we look good!

Because of righteousness, you have a relationship with the God who spoke food into existence. You have a personal relationship with Jesus, who took an ordinary meal of five loaves and two fish and fed 5,000 plus people, all with varying individual nutritional needs. This is the same God who compressed time to turn water into wine. He controls the food. And He still has the same authority over your food. You are entitled to be nourished and well-fed. You do not deserve to struggle and battle with food. But when you don't know what you are entitled to, you take whatever you can get. Don't add to what God said about food as Eve did. It is supposed to be simple even though the world makes it complicated. Your sin debt has already been paid in full. That sin debt included Adam's struggle with food. Because of Jesus, you are supposed to operate in rest.

Righteousness simply means being in right standing with God. When Adam was created, he was already righteous. Nothing was keeping Adam and God apart. When sin entered the world, God couldn't tolerate it. He couldn't even look at it. As such, Adam and God had to part. When God says we are righteous, He is saying we are innocent. He doesn't see our sins, and we no longer have a sin debt. Remember, part of the sin debt was a changed relationship with food in which it was entirely up to Adam's effort and toil. God, in His mercy, changed all of that when Jesus died on the cross. Because He made us righteous, we are no longer impacted by the consequences of the sin debt. And yet He doesn't require us to be perfect. We just need to know we are the righteousness of God in Christ Jesus. We benefit from Jesus's perfection.

Our perfection is not a requirement or even a component of righteousness. We are righteous only because of Christ Jesus. In Romans 3:24, we read, "Yet God, with undeserved kindness, declares that we are righteous. He did this through Christ Jesus when he freed us from the penalty of our sins." So, what does righteousness entitle us to when it comes to food?

There is an exciting connection between righteousness and food. It can be found in Matthew 6:31-33. "Therefore, do not worry, saying 'What shall we eat?' or 'What shall we drink?' or 'What shall we wear?' For after all these things the Gentiles seek. For your heavenly Father knows that you need all these things. But seek first the kingdom of God and His righteousness, and all these things shall be added to you." I have heard it preached that the mention of food, drink, and clothing is just provided to indicate that God will meet even our basic needs. And I believe that to be true. I also think that the Bible was written to be interpreted and understood on many different levels. We are all at different walks of the Christian life. To some who are new to a relationship with Christ, the Word is like milk for a baby. It is easy to understand taken at face value. As the relationship with the Lord deepens, then deeper nourishment is needed. Deeper analysis of a verse that had previously been milk becomes meat. The Lord gives greater insight into that verse's application for that individual. It's the same here. We can analyze the "what shall we eat" part, but taken at its basic level, how many times have you asked that very question: "What am I supposed to eat?" We try to follow the rules of a diet. We try to follow the rules or guidelines of an authority. Here, I believe that the Lord is reminding us of the advantage we have when we recognize or realize the gift of His righteousness. When you focus on that gift, because of the blood-bought relationship, He will guide you individually as to what to eat. He will add all those things to you.

For example, let's say that you keep getting a feeling that you should stop eating sugar. You hear the advice all over television. Your doctor is telling you the same thing. But most importantly, you keep getting "a feeling" that it's time for you to make a change. While you feel the thought simply is dreadful and frightening, if God is putting that on your heart, then He knows what's happening on a level that maybe you are unaware.

Furthermore, He is not going to prompt you to do something that He has not already equipped you to do. In a relationship with Him, He will guide your path. When you get prompted, and you recognize it's from Him, no matter how many times you've rebuked it or yelled, "Get behind me Satan!" because of your right-standing with Him, He has provided a fresh anointing for that time and that prompting. He's not going to let you go it alone. He knows your struggle. He's seen how many times you have tried to do this and failed on your own. He wants you to rely on Him. He will strengthen you and has promised that you can do all things through Him. Remember, you're entitled to this advantage or guarantee of success.

As we see in Matthew, what you eat matters to Him. He is telling you to give it over to Him. Let Him direct you. Stop listening to conflicting and confusing rules. Stop trying to force things to happen. You seek first His righteousness, and He will take care of all the other "things." Notice, the "things" will be added. Typically, when you diet, it's about taking things away. Seek Him first, and it will deepen your relationship with Him. He will add to you all the "things" you need to be successful.

As Christians, we have an advantage. I know that it's hard to boldly say, "I am the righteousness of God in Christ Jesus" when you feel like all you do is make dieting and food choice mistakes. We have all been hit over the head with the "your body is a temple" speech trying to guilt or force you into changes. But that is trying to do it on your own. You can't become righteous on your own. It's your belief in Jesus that made you righteous. So why should you approach your food separate and apart from Him? Self-effort will always be limited and will still run out. But the benefits of your righteousness have no limits. Tap into it. It's already yours.

So be entitled. What does righteousness allow you? To not worry about what you are going to eat. Because you are in right standing with the Food-Maker and your Creator, you have the inside scoop. Draw closer to Him. Stand confidently in your status as righteous no matter how many times you failed to diet. The Israelites repeatedly failed in keeping the Ten Commandments. The Kingdom of God is not about laws and self-effort. It's merely about righteousness and the sweet relationship with Jesus that comes from it.

When you begin to recognize the full application that you are in right standing with God, you will stop struggling with food. Adam didn't struggle until he sinned. Jesus's death on the cross paid the sin debt in full. That means there's no need for you to struggle anymore. Your success with food isn't about how much more you need to learn. It's resting and relying on the clear prompting from your Great Physician. It's knowing and declaring, "I don't have to ask, 'what should I eat?'" because "I am the righteousness of God in Christ Jesus." Now, this is not a green light to eat whatever you want. There's an industry out there capitalizing on your need for convenience. Your entitlement is an invitation to slow down and listen to God, directing you regarding how to feed yourself. The way you eat may look different than another person. But just like feeding the 5,000, everyone had different needs, but He quickly and easily took care of everyone.

God has promised that because you are righteous, you will be successful. In Romans 5:17, we read, "those who receive ... the gift of righteousness will reign in life through the One, Jesus Christ." You will reign over food controlling your life. You will reign over the addictions and food cravings that cause you to eat what you know you shouldn't. You will no longer diet; instead, you will be directed to a healthy way of eating that is suited for you. No longer will you be a slave to your food or the latest diet fad. Instead, you will be in control because He will be guiding your steps. He may guide you to Keto, Weight Watchers, or any other eating program. When He is in the middle of it, and you know He is guiding your steps, you will have success.

Every instance that you declare you are the righteousness of God in Christ Jesus, you are magnifying Jesus's death on the cross. You are reminding yourself of who you are, who you belong to, and what righteousness entitles you to have.

When we are consumed with thinking about our food, it takes away the focus from our righteousness. Romans 14:17 tells us, "For the kingdom of God is not eating and drinking, but righteousness, peace, and joy in the Holy Spirit." Our culture is obsessed with food and the negative consequences of its consumption. We are all seeking the perfect diet to get the results we want. It is easy to get caught up in it when it is being advertised to you in some form or fashion 24/7/365. Dr. Hyman reports, "Over the next 35 years, it's going to cost the US a whopping 95 trillion dollars to deal with diseases that can be prevented by lifestyle and dietary choices." When you read information like this, it is very motivating to want to make changes. But what change? Who do you listen to? What diet do you eat? You can easily get overwhelmed in the questions and answers. Instead, go to the Source. He doesn't change. He knows your body and your needs better than you do.

When you begin wondering about what to eat, seek first the kingdom of God and His righteousness. Stand on your entitlement. Trust that God will give you the information you need for your body. Plant yourself firmly on the truth that you have been given the gift of righteousness through Christ.

When you are at rest in that truth, you can sense the Lord's guidance. You have a relationship with Him that allows Him to direct your paths and your choices. Will the advice always be easy? Not necessarily. But it will be doable with His strength.

Years ago, I attended a home Bible study with members of a church I attended at the time. The concept was that a small group of church members would gather every week at someone's house to study God's Word. A byproduct of that gathering was that new relationships would develop as people studied together. One night, we were discussing the topic of righteousness. One of the members of the group happened to be an associate pastor of the church. He was leading the study and discussing how a person becomes righteous. He went around the room and had each participant state if they felt that righteousness was obtained by works or by faith.

You were to say that you were a "do-er" or a "be-er." Many people believed that they were a "do-er" in that they needed to do good things to be righteous. Some, though significantly fewer, thought they were a "be-er." The discussion then tripped into ways to become righteous such as doing charity work, being kind to people, and helping those in need. Feeling a bit troubled and confused at the perspective of the discussion, I asked the associate pastor about Genesis 15:6, which states, "Abraham believed in the Lord; and he counted it to him for righteousness." I contributed that God considered Abraham righteous simply because he believed in God. He had faith. Not because of any works that Abraham performed. He didn't earn his righteousness. Believing in

God was all it took since the death of Jesus hadn't occurred yet. The associate pastor listened attentively then replied rather abruptly, "No. You're wrong. That's the old way of thinking." After the initial shock wore off, I picked up somewhere in his response hearing him say, "There's been a great deal of debate recently as to who the pronouns "he" and "him" in "he credited it to him as righteousness" was referring, God or Abraham." I then asked, "Why would God need to be credited with righteousness? He never sinned." The associate pastor's quick reply was, "Yeah, ok. But that's the old way of thinking."

No one in the room contributed anything further to the topic. To tell you the truth, I was so shocked that I don't even remember anything more of the study. My heart was broken for those that heard the discussion and walked away, believing righteousness was something you earned by being a "do-er." When we are preoccupied with always having to do more or do better, we get exhausted, frustrated, and, as a result, we quit. It's too hard. How do you know when you've done enough to qualify for righteousness? We weren't designed for that kind of labor-intensive endurance. If we are on a constant quest to make ourselves righteous, then we miss the point of Jesus's death on the cross. Not to mention, if we must add to what Jesus accomplished on the cross, then He didn't need to die. In Romans 3:22, "We are made right with God by placing our faith in Jesus Christ. And this is true for everyone who believes, no matter who we are."

In Romans 10:10, we read, "For with the heart, man believeth unto righteousness." I believe that the relationship with Jesus will change our relationship with food. It's no longer about struggle or trial and error, for that matter. It's about knowing who you are because of the blood of Jesus. That you are entitled to benefits and advantages because the sin debt is paid in full.

Adam had a healthy relationship with food until sin entered. The ease was because of his relationship with God. Adam was close to Him; they fellowshipped. God walked in the Garden with Adam. Aside from the "don't eat from that one tree", Adam's primary instruction was to "eat freely."

The moment the sin occurred, the relationship between God and Adam was broken. It was severed because God, who is perfect and holy, cannot be in the presence of sin. Adam lost his right-standing with God. He sensed it immediately and hid from God in the Garden. He felt vulnerable, exposed, and unsafe. Adam was no longer entitled to the benefits of that relationship. The second Adam, Jesus, came and restored the connection for those who simply believe.

Because of the blood of Jesus and our robe of righteousness, God no longer sees our sins. Our sin debt is paid in full, and we are justified as if we had never sinned. Our right-standing has been restored. We can't add to it, nor can we take away from it. When Jesus said, "It is finished", it was because everything had been paid. That payment also includes our relationship to food.

So maybe the answer to all the food confusion is, along with eating real food, take advantage of the benefits you are entitled to because of righteousness. When told to "Seek first the kingdom of God and His righteousness," then "all these things shall be added unto you," what if "all these things" are health benefits that food can't provide alone? What if, because you are made righteous, then every health promise found in the Bible becomes a guarantee? People realize the consequences of not eating real food. Enough time that has passed in which a diet consisting of human-made food has created a lot of problems for a lot of people. So, what if you put your trust back in your food and body Creator? Stop looking to food to fix it; instead, look to the All-Knowing to guide you.

The advice that most people hear is based on guidelines for a national average. Whenever you have an average of something, some data points tend to be outside of that number. The advice is constructed around the scientifically researched beliefs or findings that particular foods or way of eating is beneficial for most people. But not all. For the Christian, you are not average. You were bought with a price that makes you incredibly valuable.

Furthermore, you are in the world, but you are not of the world (John 15:19 and John 17:14-16). We must be in the world because this is where we live. But we don't have to be of the world, meaning where we get our source of information.

I can picture Adam in the Garden, pulling a piece of fruit from one of the trees (all except the forbidden tree) and reclining back against the trunk, crossing his ankles. Taking his first bite, the juices of his delicious selection run down his arm. He is enjoying his food while enjoying the fellowship of the Lord sitting right there beside him as they speak. There is a closeness. Who knows, maybe they didn't even have to talk. We have that same opportunity because of the cross. Because God turned His back on His sin and sickness ridden Son, Jesus, God can never leave us or forsake us. That great exchange solidified the relationship for us. What this means is that no matter where we are, He's right there. When we are looking at the menu, God's right there. When we are standing in front of the vending machine or the grocery store, He's right there. God is ready to give us guidance that His all-knowing character is uniquely equipped to provide. To Him, we are not average. We are unique, fearfully, and wonderfully made. He knows what we need at that very moment. All we must do is ask for His guidance and be sensitive to His prompting. Could His direction go against what society is telling us to do? Absolutely! Trust Him and enjoy the benefits of the relationship that the robe of righteousness entitles you to.

In Galatians 2:16, we read, "For no one will ever be made right with God by obeying the law." It's simply not about what we do. We can never do enough to earn righteousness. Jesus's death was more than enough. We can rest in the promise of Romans 5:17 "For the sin of this one man, Adam, caused death to rule over many. But even greater is God's wonderful grace and his gift of righteousness, for all who receive it will live in triumph over sin and death through this one man, Jesus Christ." What an exciting thought to be entitled to a healthy relationship with food. There probably aren't many of us that can even imagine what that would look or feel like. For sure, the way we have approached food so far hasn't helped. Unless our perspective changes, it's only going to get worse. So be entitled! Live entitled! Wear your robe of righteousness confidently. Let it change the way you see yourself and the way you relate to your food. You are the righteousness of God through Christ Jesus, bless your heart!

CHAPTER 7

FAITH

Who would have thought that George Michael could say it best in his 1987 album title song "Faith?" For those of that generation, you already know the words: "Cause I gotta have faith. I got to have faith. Because I gotta have faith, faith, faith. I got to have faith. (Brief pause) Baby!" Ok, I'm going to stop now. I know that tune will be playing in your head for the next several hours as well. You're welcome and sorry about that. Truthfully, it's a great message. While George is telling us that he must have faith, so do we.

For the Christian, faith is vitally important. Because it activates everything, it behooves us to know what faith is. In Hebrews 11:1, we are given the definition. "Faith is the substance of things hoped for, the evidence of things not seen." I am particularly partial to Philip Yancey's description: "Faith means believing in advance what will only make sense in reverse." No matter how you define it, faith is how you see Jesus. In several of the healing accounts in the Gospels, Jesus tells the person who just received their healing, "Your faith has made you well." He didn't say it was because of the food they ate. Nor did He say it was because of how much they exercised. But instead, it was their faith in what Jesus could do for them. What are you believing your food can do for you? Are you hoping that your new diet is going to provide you with the nutrition and results to keep sickness and disease at bay? Let's unpack this for a moment. During Jesus's time on earth, people ate what is now classified as the Mediterranean diet. They also walked everywhere, typically for long distances. They also lacked the technological advances that have rendered our culture comparatively more sedentary. Yet they still needed healing. In Luke 6:19, we read of large groups of people seeking Jesus, and He "healed all who came to Him." Could it be possible that a food and exercise prescription may not be enough?

From where does faith come? According to Hebrews 12:2, it comes from Jesus. The Scripture says, "Looking unto Jesus, the author, and finisher of our faith." When we focus on Jesus and the finished work of the cross, that's faith. Faith comes from knowing what Jesus accomplished on the cross. The Bible tells us there are levels of faith.

We read that it can be the size of a mustard seed and will move a mountain. Faith is that powerful.

So how do we apply faith to our topic of food? We put a lot of emphasis on food to heal us. Conversely, we believe that food can also make us sick. Yet, the Scripture tells us that the finished work of the cross takes away all sicknesses and all diseases. Does the state of our health depend that much on food alone?

We consistently exercise faith when it comes to our diet. We have confidence that the Keto diet is going to work for us this time. We have faith that eliminating sugar is going to provide health benefits, and it will. The emphasis is typically on how we can change our way of eating to earn more exceptional health results. But we usually don't factor Jesus into the equation. There has never been a time in history where faith in our food was more prevalent. There are several other diets to attempt when the one you are currently on doesn't work. You believe there must be one that will work; you just must find it. All the advertisements tell you their diet plan is just what you need. Your friends tell you of the most recent scientific breakthrough in food research and why you should now include kale chips into your diet. We are exposed to a lot of data about food. With each new piece of information, we hope it is going to make the difference. Where is your faith placed? Is it on the "latest and greatest" or is it in Jesus?

In Romans 10:6, we read, "But the righteousness of faith speaks." When you state "I am the righteousness of God in Christ Jesus," that is exercising your faith. But faith in what? When we pin our hopes for weight loss or health recovery on our food without faith in the Food Creator or the Great Physician, we are missing the key ingredient. Because you know you are righteous, you are entitled to success. Philippians 4:13 guarantees you can do all things through Christ because He strengthens you. You get the progress or the results because He adds His "super" to your "natural" ability. The focus isn't on you and your efforts. Talk to Him about your health goals. Tell Him what you would like to accomplish. Invite Him to help you create a plan. Not only will He guide and direct you, but He will also enable you to get results.

Here is a diet challenge: take the Bible at its Word. I know the thought of totally relying on God to guide and direct your eating can make you nervous. It is unheard of to rely on such a thing.

Hebrews 11:6 tells us, "Without faith, it is impossible to please God." The eleventh chapter of Hebrews is considered the "faith chapter." It lists the "Hall of Faith" or the "Heroes of Faith" who demonstrate what a life of faith can produce. Faith, the size of a mustard seed, can move a mountain (Matthew 17:20). Place a mustard seed in the palm of your hand. More than likely, you will be looking around to see if you dropped it on the floor. It is so small that it will roll between or nestle into the cracks between your fingers. It is very tiny.

You see, the Lord is not interested in the amount of the faith. Otherwise, He would have given us a chart showing us the amount of faith needed for each miracle or request we could ever want. Instead, He is interested in where your faith is directed. Do you have faith in what His Word says? Do you have faith in the promises He has spoken to your heart? Do you have faith in His guidance regarding what you should be eating? He knows your struggle. He knows your questions and confusion. 1 Corinthians 14:33 tells us, "God is not the author of confusion." Eve succumbed to the serpent simply because she was confused. The serpent asked a question that she could not answer definitively. God has your answers, and you are entitled to them because you are the righteousness of God in Christ Jesus. When you have faith the size of a mustard seed, you can tell the mountain to be removed and it will. Something that small can contain incredible power when it contains faith. Faith is a crucial ingredient in a Christian's diet. Keep looking to the cross and identifying what Jesus's blood purchased. Jesus's blood fixed what was broken and restored that which was lost in the Garden. There was nothing left undone. Since food was a big part of the Garden, having faith in the restorative work of the cross changed man's relationship to food. But only for those who believe; for those who have faith.

Instead of the power of faith, we tend to focus on the amount of faith we have. We try to find ways to increase it. But again, that is putting the effort on ourselves. Focusing on Jesus is all that matters.

In several healing stories of the Bible, Jesus is quoted as saying, "Let it be done according to your faith." At that precise moment, the people were seeking an answer to a health issue. Jesus didn't whip out a legal pad and begin asking dietary questions. He did not care what they had eaten for breakfast. With the power of faith, it did not matter. Jesus was not hindered if someone skipped a meal. He wasn't limited because the person overate. We read of no mention of those who were seeking healing doing a dietary inventory before seeking Jesus. Regardless of why they were experiencing their physical issue, their faith that Jesus was their only answer was more than enough. They weren't just healed; they were restored. But the accurate measure was how did they see Jesus? Did they see Him as someone who may or may not heal them? Did they see Him as someone too busy to care about their family member? No. He was the solution, the missing part of all the attempts they had made before their encounter with Him. It was their faith. Was Jesus willing? Yes. Was Jesus capable? Absolutely. Is Jesus still willing and capable? You bet. Can and will Jesus guide you in how to eat? Most definitely. When we get sick, we turn to our food. The first place we should turn is Jesus. Knowing what the Bible says about food, Jesus, and the cross will serve to deepen your understanding and your faith in Jehovah Rapha, your Healer.

It would be different if somewhere in the Bible, we are told of food's connection to specific diseases. I have not found it. So, what we can firmly stand on and attach our faith to is that Jesus's blood removed the curse on the ground. Jesus's death on the cross took away the struggle and toil to find or make bread. Jesus's blood at the whipping post and His death on the cross provided healing and removed every sickness and disease. Do you have faith that you are justified? It is "just as if" you had never sinned. If it is as if you've never sinned, then it's as if you have no punishment. Christians are living with consequences that do not belong to them anymore, and there's nothing for you to pay. The relationship with food before Adam and Eve's disobedience was to "eat freely." So, for those who have been purchased with the blood of Jesus, shouldn't that still be the case?

Do you have faith that you can talk to God about your food? Because of the cross, you can. You are covered in grace and can approach Him at any moment and any time of the day. He is right there waiting for you. Do you have faith that when you pray over your food in Jesus's name, it becomes just what your body needs? Because of the cross, you can. When Jesus fed the 5,000, it became what each person in attendance required. Jesus is still the same today, and He'll be the same tomorrow (Hebrews 13:8).

In the Christmas hymn, Joy to the World, we sing in the second stanza: "Joy to the World, the Savior reigns! Let men their songs employ, while fields and floods, rocks, hills and plains, Repeat the sounding joy." When we sing this hymn, we are rejoicing over the birth of the Savior. But we are also acknowledging the impact of Jesus on the fields, rocks, hills, and plains. The earth responds to Jesus. The earth felt the effects of Jesus's birth and death because it felt the impact of God's and Adam's separation. The ground was included in the punishment. The earth was altered by sin in that the land was cursed. And since the ground produces our food, we need to know that Jesus and the earth are still connected.

How does one function in faith? By establishing your faith upon the promises in His Word. Everyone has faith in something. Even if you are not cognizant of what it is. You have faith that the sun will rise tomorrow morning. You know this because you do not have to think about it every night before you go to bed. You can also have faith that something terrible will happen. How do you know that? You consistently worry about it. You know it is coming, and you're just waiting for it. How you use your faith is worth considering. Faith can become a habit. Establishing a habit takes brain energy. You must identify what it is you are staking your faith to. For our purposes here, develop your faith in the relationship God wants you to have with your food. And it starts with Jesus and the cross.

Faith comes by hearing and hearing by the word of Christ (Romans 10:17). The more you understand His perspective of food, the more you believe what He says. Your faith will continue to grow. There are no limits to how tremendous your faith can be. For the Christian, developing your faith in a specific area takes hearing. I encourage you to take some time to focus on what you have been hearing. We are bombarded with information on an hourly basis. More accurately, with the internet and social media, minute by minute. If you are routinely feeding on information connecting food and health, then that is where your faith will grow. Again, I am not saying that food does not have that kind of power. I believe it does. But bring Jesus into the picture. Can He do more for you than food can? Yes. Your food and Jesus are not mutually exclusive. Jesus can supersede the impact of food.

The topic of food is not so insignificant to God that we can't apply faith to it. Quite the contrary. It is a decision that most of us must make at least three times a day. Yet we give it little thought or consideration. We grab food "on the go" running out the door to the busy day awaiting us. We then eat at our desk during lunch or mindlessly inhale a meal while working on other projects. We arrive home exhausted with little to no energy or interest in cooking. Understandably, it is easier to have dinner delivered. Since God designed us to need food, talk to Him about your routine. Ask Him to help you make adjustments that will benefit you and your family. He is patiently waiting.

When we exercise our faith, it means believing and speaking the promises found in His Word.

The Bible provides us a solid foundation. When we stake our faith to a firm foundation, we know that it will never change. What God says about food is always the same. Compare that to placing our trust in the government recommendations and doctors' advice. How many times have you felt frustrated because the rules or suggestions changed? A few years ago, eggs were blamed for raising a person's cholesterol and fast-tracking them to heart disease. Today, according to Healthline.com, eggs are "linked to a reduced risk of heart disease."[1]

In a few years, who knows what the "experts" will tell us? We see this advice vacillating in connection with many of our foods, and this is the reason many people stop paying attention. Do you have faith in what the authorities tell you?

You have been burned. You have redesigned your lifestyle to accommodate the new recommendations only to find that they weren't as correct as they thought. A new study came along, completely changing the advice you were given. Everyone wants to put their faith in something sure. Something solid. If the ground on which you are standing continues to shift, then you do not have a lot of confidence that it can support you.

That is a healthy and natural response. How do you put your faith in something that is always changing? Eventually, you develop faith in the fact that it will change. Then you do not pay attention or care anymore. But God's Word never changes. Nor does He. His instructions are always the same.

God is not biased. His instruction comes from a place of love with no thought of what He can get from it. Compare that to the food industry giants who are solely interested in competition and making a profit. Michael Moss reported on this very mindset and motivation of the Coca Cola company. I am not saying that food industry leaders are out to hurt people. I would like to believe that they're not. Their responsibility is to their Board members and stockholders who expect the company to make a profit. Moss writes about Jeffrey Dunn, a past CEO of the Coca-Cola Company.

"In pursuing this massive consumption, Dunn rose nearly to the top of the company. He became president for North and South America, a job that entailed winning the brand loyalty of nine hundred million people. He lived Coke and loved his work and the company, a devotion shared by many at Coke, and for all those years, he had no qualms about what he sold. He achieved this peace of mind, he said, by simply not thinking about what he sold.

'At Coke, I do think they believe they are doing the right things,' he said. If you really think you are doing the wrong thing and covering it up, it's hard to deal with that emotionally. I've still got friends there, and I suggest to them, 'It's just extremely hard to see yourself from the inside.'"

"But you can look at the obesity rates, and you can look at per capita consumption of sugary soft drinks and overlay those on a map, and I promise you: They correlate about 99. 999 percent. As they say, you can run, but you can't hide."

These companies are driven to make a profit. Good business practice requires them to do so to stay in business and to employ thousands of people. It's no different for a car company or a mattress company. Without profit, there is no business. The food items produced by the industry are deemed "safe" for public consumption by the government. They say their products do not hurt people. So, if you just pay attention to the motivation, are you putting your faith in the for-profit company, the Food and Drug Administration, and in the Federal Trade Commission?

The information provided to us as consumers is very confusing. The companies have admitted to fostering brand loyalty at younger ages so that they have waves of new customers every generation. Children are marketed to with a plan to create loyal and addicted soft drink consumers by the time they reach the age of twelve. According to Moss, Coke's research showed that 12-year-old children begin earning an allowance. With that money, they visit convenience stores and are exercising some independence in their food and drink consumption. This demographic is strategically targeted so that they will be "loyal brand customers" when they get older. When we depend on man swayed by profit, bias, and competition to direct our food consumption choices, the result is always confusion. Remember, the Bible says in 1 Corinthians 14:33, "For God is not the author of confusion." Sadly, the food industry admittedly uses schemes and manipulation to entice and addict a person to keep purchasing and eating their food. They want and need loyal consumers so that their company remains competitive and ideally number one. These companies are not selling nutrition and health. They are not even selling food. They are providing a product to the marketplace. Just as with any other consumable product, the consumer has a choice. The company knows it and uses clever marketing tools to influence that choice.

Compare that to the simplicity of real food. God created it for man's consumption with the divine marketing message: "eat freely." There are no complicated labels to interpret. There are no warnings. Between these two options, where is your faith?

Part of our challenge is that we see food as only providing a physical benefit. But for the Christian, I believe an awareness of the spiritual impact is missing. Real food was created from the voice of God. He commanded the ground to produce plants. The animals He provided as our food also eat the plants He created. From that same ground, He lovingly fashioned man. Whenever we eat God-created food, aside from the nutrients, I believe that there are spiritual elements and benefits. This food is alive and responsive to the voice of God.

A classic Bible story of faith occurred in Matthew 8:26 that tells of the disciples and Jesus in a boat sailing to the Gadarenes. While Jesus was asleep, a storm developed. The disciples panicked, believing that their boat was going to capsize. They woke Jesus. Verse 26 tells us, "He replied, 'You of little faith, why are you so afraid?' Then He got up and rebuked the winds and the waves, and it was completely calm." Notice the first thing that He points out to the disciples is that they had little faith. The overwhelming and frightening external stimuli bombarded them even with Jesus in the boat. In their panic, they failed to consider that Jesus controlled nature. He demonstrated His control with a straightforward rebuke to the wind. Amid a powerful storm, He was pointing out that the essential element in the situation was their faith in Him. Similarly, we get overwhelmed by our external environment. We are pelted with information that tells us something contrary to the Word. We lose our footing. We panic. For many people, there is a real fear of getting sick or dying. For the disciples in the boat, the answer was right there with them all along. Jesus didn't pay attention to the external environment. Why? It didn't affect Him. It is the same for us. If we can stop focusing on the external advice of authorities and instead put our faith in the answer that is right there in our lifeboat with us, then things can and will calm down. Do not have little faith when it comes to your food. Instead, have unshakeable faith when it comes to Jesus. Ephesians 4:14 tells us, "Then we will no longer be infants, tossed back and forth by the waves, and blown here and there by every wind of teaching and by the cunning and craftiness of people in their deceitful scheming." I found this verse to be applicable to what we experience with our food. We are bombarded by messages and promises that certain foods are going to make us healthy and help us lose weight. Additionally, the environment our food is grown in has changed so much and is out of our control. The food industry has introduced Roundup, genetically modified foods, and toxins into our food supply, all of which are harmful. On our own, we are helpless to fight that battle. We have little control over how our food is produced. But we have the promise in Isaiah 54:17 that nothing formed against us will prosper. And in Psalm 118:6, "The Lord is my helper; I will not fear; what can man do to me?"

Do we put our faith in food to fight disease when Jesus took away all sickness and disease? Do we put our faith in food to keep us looking young when He promises in Psalm 1:3 that your leaf will not wither? Looking to food alone is the world's way of thinking. We have assigned responsibility to food to do things that Jesus has already done for us on the cross. We eat specific foods based on the health benefits we expect to get from them. For example, it is reported that pistachios reduce cholesterol and blood pressure. Bananas may help leukemia cells from growing. Avocados can prevent osteoporosis. Now, eggs are linked to a reduced risk of heart disease. You can spend an entire day researching the Internet for a list of health benefits of any and all foods you eat. Anytime you consume a food in connection with an illness or a disease, that food functions as a drug. Foods that God made do indeed have health benefits. Do any of us have the time to remember which food we are supposed to take for which disease? Jesus made it simple. Eat freely. He took away all sickness and disease on the cross.

When the sole focus of Christianity is the forgiveness of our sins and spending eternity in heaven, we miss a crucial and vital application of the Word to our daily lives. Did you even know you can have faith regarding what you eat? That, in the Bible, there is no specific diet recommended? There's Jesus and what He did at the cross.

According to God's declaration in Genesis, food is supposed to be "pleasing and good to the sight." James 1:17 tells us that whatever is good and perfect is a gift from God. He created food in the Garden and then called it "good." He did not call it "good enough," nor did He say, "Eh, that'll do for now."

Even when eating "healthy," how do you know it is the right food for you? How do you know that it will keep you from getting sick or feeling bad? There are countless stories of people who were incredibly careful about their diet but died suddenly or developed a sickness. You know those stories. And each one causes us a bit of concern. In response, typically, someone who is not interested in eating healthy will say, "See, I knew eating leaves would kill ya!" Admittedly, it makes you think for a moment. The world has made food complicated because there are so many things we expect it to do. Think of all the things to consider: is your food the correct balance of protein, carbohydrates, and fat? Does what you eat contain the right number of calories for your activity level, is your food organic? How many times should you eat a day, two, three, or six? Should everyone have to do a math equation to feed themselves with the correct grams of each macronutrient? We hear that if you eat too many calories, your body stores what it does not use as the dreaded, unwanted fat. Even studying nutrition for many years, my head is swimming just thinking about it.

We put a lot of faith in our physicians. We expect that, after years of medical school, they know what our bodies need. Doctors are wonderful. They are trained in handling medical crises and health issues. Thankfully, with the use of medication, they can slow down a disease process before it gets too far. But we also have a Great Physician. We consult with Him when we or a loved one become sick. Sadly, most of us think He is too busy to care about how we feed ourselves. I like that God refers to Himself as the Great Physician as opposed to the Greatest Physician. Using the comparative form of the adjective "great" indicates that there's God, then there are all the other physicians in a separate group. Not that they are not highly qualified physicians or that they are not experts at what they do. They just aren't at the level of the Great Physician. We look to our physicians to give us nutrition advice. But we have a Great Physician who designed the food and the body that needs it. And food is God's gift. The Bible tells us, "Man does not live by bread alone." I believe what He is saying is that food is not the total answer. We have assigned a lot of responsibility and blame onto food when we are not eating food at all or at least not based on the Lord's definition. Man can never create food-like products that are nutritionally equal or superior to what God has already made.

Michael Moss continued his report into Coke's targeting twelve years old kids. He reports that one of the executives admitted, "'Magically when they would turn twelve, we'd suddenly attack them like a bunch of wolves,' said Putman. Starting at twelve, kids have more allowance to spend, travel to and from school on their own, and often leave the school grounds for lunch. Most critically, they begin to form the likes and dislikes that will define them for the rest of their lives. Coke studied these metrics, of course, and planned its campaigns accordingly."

However, the company directed much of its marketing effort at young adults to sustain and grow consumption rates. Moss explains that "the Coca-Cola Retailing Research Council ... plumbs the social science of shopping to identify the ways in which both teens and adults can be made more vulnerable to persuasion."

Again, I am not here to denigrate the food industry. The industry has a job to do, and it does it well. However, the more I learn, the more I find the information upsetting. Authors who have studied the industry and reported their findings tend to use terms such as "manipulation," "scheme," "deception," "lies," and "profit." We must take the industry at face value. And stop seeing them as a source of healthy food. What is their motivation? By their own admission, it's not our health. Their job is to push a product and make a profit to satisfy their board members and stockholders. It is a business and a burgeoning, competitive one at that. They are jockeying and vying for consumers' limited food dollars. People want it cheap; they want it convenient, and they want it tasty. The industry is all too willing to comply and meet that demand.

Back to the original question: Where is your faith? Is it misplaced? Do you have faith that the people who "make" food are interested in your health? Do you believe that making the correct food choices makes the difference between sickness and health? If your body is designed to run on real food, and the cross took away every sickness and disease, then shouldn't this be where your faith is tethered? Put your faith in Jesus. Let your faith make you well.

Romans Chapter 14 describes the influence of faith in connection with the food a person chooses to eat. We read, "One man's faith allows him to eat everything, but another man, whose faith is weak, eats only vegetables. The man who eats everything must not look down on him who does not, and the man who does not eat everything must not condemn the man who does, for God has accepted him. . . He who eats meat, eats to the Lord, for he gives thanks to God; and he who abstains, does so to the Lord and gives thanks to God. ... As one who is in the Lord Jesus, I am fully convinced that no food is unclean in itself. But if anyone regards something as unclean, then for him it is unclean. For the kingdom of God is not a matter of eating and drinking, but of righteousness, peace and joy in the Holy Spirit.

So, whatever you believe about these things keep between yourself and God. Blessed is the man who does not condemn himself by what he approves. But the man who has doubts is condemned if he eats, because his eating is not from faith; and everything that does not come from faith is sin."

This long passage demonstrates that what you eat is between you and the Lord. It is based on your faith. Take the time to talk to Him and let His perspective about food begin to mold and shape yours.

In 2 Corinthians 5:7, we are told to "Live by faith, not by sight." When we eat, we cannot see what is happening to the food on the inside of our bodies. But by faith, we can believe it is nourishing us. God created it and has promised that, as our Shepherd, we will not lack anything. In Psalm 84:11, we read, "No good thing will He withhold from those who walk uprightly." When He created food, He said it was good. He promises to make sure we have what we need.

In James 2:26, we are told: "Faith without works is dead." Faith is not enough. We must put action to our faith. We can have faith that Jesus changed our relationship to food. He is not telling us that we must work to make the food better for us. Nor is this verse an invitation for self-effort. Instead, we can work to develop our faith when we eat the food coupled with a greater understanding of Jesus and the cross. Together, the results are transformative.

Bob Goff, author of the New York Times bestselling book *Love Does*, is quoted, "We're following a God we can't see, for a lifetime we can't measure, to an eternity we can't comprehend, because of grace we didn't earn. Faith isn't a bunch of facts." When we exercise our faith in connection with our diet, food is not about a "bunch of facts" either. It is about Jesus.

According to Mark Batterson in his book *In a Pit with a Lion on a Snowy Day*, "Faith gives us the dimensional freedom to overcome our human limitations by exiting space-time via prayer." He continues, "How you think about God will determine who you become. And that internal picture of God determines how you see everything else." I believe how you see God determines your relationship with food. Mark adds, "Long before God laid earth's foundations, He had us in mind. He thought of everything, provided for everything we could possibly need." We see this in God's preparation of the Garden. In His excited anticipation of Adam's arrival, He included food. God is still that interested and passionate about your food. You just "gotta have faith."

CHAPTER 8

PEACE

My peace I leave with you. What is peace? We hear the word in conjunction with the phrase "Peace in the Middle East" or "Peace on Earth" at Christmas time. To our understanding, peace seems temporary or something we need to find or obtain. It is a fleeting condition or state of being. Truthfully, do we ever expect peace in the Middle East or on earth? The term "peace" gets bantered around with little expectation of it becoming a reality. But when Adam walked in the Garden with God, he did so in a state of peace, both externally and internally. A peaceful environment and mental state were Adam's reality.

According to *Baker's Evangelical Dictionary of Biblical Theology*, the word peace stems from the root word shalom, which means "to be complete or to be sound." The Dictionary continues to explain that the noun form has many "nuances but can be grouped into categories." In part, peace or shalom means "wholeness of life or body (i.e., health); a right relationship or harmony between two parties or people" as well as "prosperity, success, or fulfillment." When it comes to the relationship with food, all three categories are important. First, though out of definitional order, we have a right relationship with God because of the cross. There is harmony between God and us, just as there was with Adam in the Garden.

Second, we are physically made whole. Most of us are on a constant quest to fix what is missing or broken in our bodies. We are searching for ways to avoid getting sick or developing a chronic illness. And we are painfully aware when things just are not working right. When illness is present, we are not whole. In nutrition circles, the word "disease" is described as "dis-ease" or lack of ease. It is true. There is an absence of vitality; we are missing health. The only place we are taught to look to regain our health is our food or the medications prescribed by a physician. But God is the single source for perfect wholeness. Not only can He fix the issue, He can restore wholeness so that we are even better than before.

Third, with peace, we have success in all we do. This includes our food-related goals. Whatever the motivation, we all come to a place in life where we want to eat right or at least make better choices. It is so commonplace that we do not even realize how much it consumes our thoughts. Some people want to lose weight. Some people need to gain weight. Some need to develop a more positive relationship with food. To compete in bodybuilding competitions, people manipulate their nutrient composition to alter their body composition.

No matter the physical goal, it seems that everything can be traced back to the topic of food. But with peace, God's peace, we are guaranteed to have success. Nothing is missing or broken. Can you imagine?

Another helpful definition of peace is "a stress-free state of security or calmness." That would be nice. If we have been given His promise that "He will keep you in perfect peace," then why are we not all living in perfect peace? We have become accustomed to thinking that peace is transitory. It comes and goes. We tend to believe it is present in the good days and absent in the bad days. On good days there is more peace; we're happier. Peace is something to hope or strive for, but it can be lost easily.

According to Wikipedia, "Shalom is a Hebrew word meaning peace, harmony, wholeness, completeness, prosperity, welfare and tranquility and can be used idiomatically to mean both hello and goodbye." The sheer fact that shalom is used as both a greeting and parting word implies that it is not a permanent state. It must be reestablished frequently.

In Judges 6:24, we read that God is the "Source of Peace." This is not just any peace; it is perfect peace. Any other peace obtained by man's efforts is an inferior substitute. Perfect peace carries with it the promise of permanence. Regular, run-of-the-mill peace is fleeting and short-lived. It must be maintained by repeated work; otherwise, the peace is lost.

In Isaiah 26:3 and 2 Thessalonians 3:16, we read, "You will keep in perfect peace all who trust in you, all whose thoughts are fixed on you." Notice, for the Christian, who is doing the work? God is the one who keeps us in peace. And not just any old peace but "perfect peace." All other peace by nature is imperfect. It fails. It tires out. We tire out and do not invest the effort to maintain it. By the definitions used above, when we operate in peace, we have health. The problem is that we tend to manufacture our peace through a variety of ineffective means. We meditate. We get massages. These activities are wonderful, but the benefits are temporary. And they do not result in a lasting peace.

God wants us to trust Him with our food and eating habits. He wants us to know what He has said about food. Stop putting our trust in all the conflicting authority that keeps up frustrated and confused. When we trust in Him, we have perfect peace.

We have a right relationship with God because of the cross. Peace is an automatic byproduct of Jesus's death. When we start looking at everything around us competing for our attention, we can lose our peace. When this happens, it is easy to take our eyes off God. When we focus on God as we are making decisions for our food and health, and we include Him in the decision-making process, we will have peace that we are making the right choices for ourselves.

We cannot manufacture perfect peace. It is not a byproduct of our efforts. It is a God-given gift to the Christian. Yet, failing to recognize that we have it, that we are entitled to it, or that it was purchased for us, can have negative consequences. We live our lives without it, and we then search for inferior peace substitutes in and from other places.

In the Garden, Adam was in a peaceful environment. It

was not peaceful because it was always the perfect temperature and humidity. Or because the sun shone every day, and the birds were always singing. While this sounds like peace to us the external environment had nothing to do with it. What created peace was Adam's relationship to God. There was no strife. Adam was secure in his relationship with his Creator. God and Adam spent time together, and they talked often. Naturally, because Adam had not experienced anything but peace, Adam couldn't imagine a world without it. Lack of peace is not possible in the presence of God. Sadly, and to the contrary, we cannot imagine a world with lasting peace. Peace was Adam's normal until he ate the forbidden fruit. As soon as his pearly whites sunk into the fantastic flesh of that forbidden fruit, the perfect peace was gone. As a result, both Adam and Eve hid because they were afraid. Genesis 3:10 tells that Adam said to God, "I heard Your voice in the garden, and I was afraid because I was naked; and I hid myself." It is worth noting the contrast. Adam admitted to God that he was afraid. In the New Testament, God, who sees us through the blood of Jesus, repeatedly tells us to "Fear not." In God's heartbrokenness, though He may have wanted to say those exact words to Adam, He could not because of the presence of sin.

Adam's confession is the first time the word "afraid" is used in the Bible. Adam felt this fear because he had lost his peace. In other words, he lost his connection with God. It was the first time he experienced distance and separation. His entire world was turned upside down. Imagine the jarring smack of Adam's new reality the moment perfect peace was gone. We are keenly aware of when we cycle in and out of peace. The lack of peace is a signal that something is just not right. But for Adam, I imagine it provided quite a wallop. Simultaneously, Adam had to grapple with a new sense of exposure and vulnerability. Without God's presence, he was indeed on his own. And he sensed the loss. Everything was up to him now. The nakedness he was aware of was an unarticulated need for the robe of righteousness that Jesus would bring. As a woefully insufficient substitute, Adam and Eve covered themselves with fig leaves. Self-effort was now their reality. But the Lord, in His love and grace, covered them with animal skin, which was a temporary solution foreshadowing the death of Jesus.

In a relationship with Jesus, He tells us, "Do not worry about your life, what you will eat or what you will drink; nor about your body." We find this in Matthew 6:25. That is not to say that you neglect these topics entirely or leave them to "chance." Our bodies are considered temples of the Holy Ghost. The point is God does not want you constantly worrying if you are doing the right thing, nor does He want you putting the state of your health squarely on what you eat. He tells us to "Cast all your anxiety on him because he cares for you" (1 Peter 5:7). Do not carry the burden yourself. When we do, we are not in peace. We were not designed to carry stress. With God, He wants to do the heavy lifting. In exchange, He invites us to come alongside Him and bear the light end of the load. He says in Matthew 11:30, "My yoke is easy and my burden is light."

It is easy to worry about what to eat when you are trying

to navigate the labyrinth of information bombarding you at any given moment. Sometimes it helps to know the motivation of the source behind the advice or recommendation. For example, the food industry will tell you that it is ok to eat processed foods. Still, according to Moss, "scientists said they could find no level of consumption of processed meats that were safe. Every 1. 7 ounces of processed meats consumed per day increased the risk of colorectal cancer by 21 percent." Yikes! In response to the scientific opinion above, the beef industry launched "a massive preemptive strike to undermine – and, if possible, discredit – the scientists' report before it reached the American people." The industry used $1. 2 million in part and "retained the services of a consulting firm called Exponent, which provides expert witnesses to industrial clients under legal duress." With the use of analytical firms, which evaluated media coverage of the beef industry, and the resulting focus group pinpointing consumers greatest concerns regarding diet and nutrition, "they prepared stores to give beef friendly media outlets" and chose "ones that were likely to produce the warmest feelings for beef among consumers." The result was that "the blows from the cancer report were significantly softened by the industry's counter programming." These are people we are supposed to believe and trust with our diet.

In perfect peace, we do not have to worry about who is telling us what. It doesn't matter because we have a relationship with Jesus, who, according to John 16:13, "will guide you into all truth." That is all any of us want. Just tell us the truth about the food we are eating. We can make informed decisions if we have the information. But as Christians, we can take it one step further. We don't have to know everything because God does. He wants to guide and direct your path. We have been so focused on what the experts tell us that we have not paid much attention to what the food-Creator has to say. He knows what is right for you and what isn't regardless of what the "experts" say.

When we refer to peace concerning food, based on the above definition, we can expect health and success. Not because of the knowledge we have accumulated. Not because of our works. And not because we successfully stayed on the cabbage diet for six weeks. Instead, it is because of the relationship with God made possible by Jesus's death on the cross. Adam lost his peace in the Garden. Before that, he never worried about food. Eve did not even fear that she was gaining weight. That is an accurate measure of peace! Jesus' death has given back to us the perfect peace we are really craving.

Fear, anxiety, and stress are all possible in the absence of peace. Remember, peace isn't the environment. Peace is internal. We can't force peace. We just need to know where to find it. But a word of caution is that we can, however, lose our peace when we take our eyes off Jesus. It is so easy to do when you have just heard a medical report or commercial warning about eating meat or eggs, for example. Or, when you've read about a study in which everyone needs to lower their cholesterol even more. Do not lose your peace. Do just like Adam did in the Garden and talk to the Lord.

In Genesis 3:17, God tells Adam the reason for the

punishment was "Because you listened to your wife and ate the fruit from the tree about which I commanded you, 'You must not eat it.'" He then doles out the sad, harsh ramifications. He is telling Adam that he is in the situation because he listened to someone who did not have their facts straight. Very clearly and very simply, God said, "Eat this, not that." When we listen to "authorities" who tell us what is safe for us to eat, we need to know the motive. The food industry motive is profit and loyal consumers. They do not hide this fact. They have hired chemists, scientists, marketers, and lobbyists, to provide you with food that appears healthy to eat. They are motivated by competition, market share, job security, and promotion. Once the daughter of Lunchables creator, Bob Drane, realized what ingredients comprised the prepacked, processed food, she criticized and questioned the integrity of her father. She could not understand how a person could create such an unhealthy item for innocent people's consumption. She reported to Moss, "For him, it was an effort to create jobs in [the] community... He also saw it from a cultural standpoint, that there was a need for something like a Lunchable for people who didn't have the resources I have. And maybe the outcome was not the most desirable product, but the impulse was right."

The individuals employed by or involved in the food industry are not out to poison people. The industry does not view it as their responsibility to nourish you. Instead, they simply cater to your need for convenience and their need to keep their jobs. These are the truths that must be accepted.

Geoffrey Bible, the former CEO of Philip Morris, stated

when it comes to processed food, "People could point to these things and say 'They have got too much sugar, they've got too much salt. Well, that is what the customer wants, and we're not putting a gun to their head to eat it. That is what they want. If we give them less, they will buy less, and the competitor will get our market.'"

So, just like Adam and Eve, who are you listening to? When either listened to the wrong person, it cost them their peace. Are you listening to the Source of truth? Are you letting the Source of your perfect peace guide and direct your food steps?

Without peace, and under stress, the relationship with food changes. We see this in Adam's situation. Separated from God, Adam had to struggle for his food. He had to rely on self-effort.

The Bible tells us to "Be anxious for nothing." This is a command, not advice. This is not the same as when a friend tells you, "don't worry about it." With God, it is different. He does not want us to hide or isolate ourselves in our fear or stress. He knows the physical consequences and the toll it can take on our bodies. Plus, when God says, "Be anxious for nothing," it is because He has already taken care of the something we're worried about. He means it. He can say that because He has the answer. God IS the answer. He does not want us worried about feeding ourselves. God wants us to benefit from the peace He purchased for us on the cross. The relationship with Him has been reestablished as if the sin and the punishment had never taken place.

There is an interesting physical and spiritual parallel

taking place the precise moment Adam and Eve ate the fruit. Because they ate from the forbidden tree, their spiritual lives were forever impacted. We all know too well that stress or lack of peace is a spiritual consequence with physical ramifications. Our bodies do not respond well to chronic stress. Once the body becomes exhausted from trying to compensate, inconvenient symptoms begin to show up.

People substitute food for many things that the Lord has promised to do for them. Food brings them short-term happiness. Eating is a form of medication. Food is supposed to provide healing if you eat the right foods. We all know of people who "eat their feelings." People use food to cover up loneliness, sadness, or low self-worth. But no matter the misuse, food is a poor substitute. It can never take the place of a genuine relationship with Him, a relationship that includes all aspects of who you are, both the good and the not-so-good. Do not worry. We all have both.

The trees in the Garden provided food that was good and pleasing to look at. Oftentimes, you will hear many of the chefs on the cooking shows talk about how you "eat with your eyes first." You know what I mean. The food might taste great, but if the presentation is not visually appealing, then you are not as likely to taste it. Growing up, whenever I wanted to cook something new, my dad was my guinea pig. I never had to ask him; it was just an understood arrangement. There were some successes. And there were some failures – significant failures. He and I still laugh at how I once tried to make pork chops in the oven, baking the foil into the meat. Dad would make sure there was a box of cereal in the cabinet just in case my new recipe did not work. We still have no clue what I did to those pork chops. Dad took one look at the shiny-flecked meat laying in the baking dish then walked over to the cereal cabinet. I went to the refrigerator and grabbed the milk. We never found out how it tasted because it looked so unappetizing. The dogs would not eat it either. Maybe dogs eat with their eyes first, too. Who knows?

Adam and Eve hid behind the trees to hide from the Lord. Think about that. Adam used a tree to stand between himself and God. Years later, God would use a tree in the form of a cross to prevent anything from ever standing between Him and man again.

We are all familiar with the 23rd Psalm. But in context with its surrounding chapters, we can see an especially important picture. Psalm 22 references the crucifixion. In verse 1 of the same chapter, the Psalmists writes, "My God, my God, why have you forsaken Me?" These are the same words Jesus cried out to His Father in the New Testament account of the crucifixion in Matthew 27:46. The 23rd chapter immediately follows this crucifixion chapter of Psalms. Here we read, "The Lord is my Shepherd. I shall not want." This relationship is possible because of the cross. In verse 2, we read that He will provide our food in "He makes me to lie down in green pastures." We, the sheep, are surrounded by our ideal food, grass. Our Father is still very much interested in our food supply and our nourishment. Notice the sheep are not running from wild animals while they are trying to eat. That would be stressful. Just the same, God wants us at peace when it comes to our food. When we rely on Him, He keeps us near our food supply and enables us to rest.

The verses of John 10:1-6 are entitled "Jesus the True Shepherd." Verses 7-21 are entitled "Jesus, the Good Shepherd," and verses 22-30 are entitled "The Shepherd Knows His Sheep." In John 10:11, Jesus declares, "I am the good shepherd. The good shepherd gives His life for the sheep." In verse 15, He states, "I lay down My life for the sheep." And that is what He did on the cross. The relationship between a shepherd and his sheep is a relevant picture. The sheep are entirely dependent upon the shepherd and symbolizes how God wants us to be with Him. When we have a relationship with Jesus, we have a relationship with the Good Shepherd. He takes care of all our needs, including our food, and He wants us to eat in peace.

The most significant indicator of a good shepherd is the condition of the sheep he is tending. Are they skinny and lethargic? Do they have tufts of wool missing? Are they limping? Or are they healthy with beautiful wool, bright eyes, and boundless energy? How the shepherd feeds his sheep matters. It's a reflection on him. Now, if the sheep wander off from the shepherd and try to find food on their own, the chances of them finding better options are slim to none. You see, the shepherd knows what the sheep need and when they need it. He knows where the best pastures and watering spots are located. The shepherd doesn't feed them in an environment where they are in danger, or where there is subpar food. He doesn't take them to a pasture full of rocks and briars. So why would the Good Shepherd do the same thing? He knows what we need. It is all about the sheep staying close to their shepherd. It is all about the relationship. Staying close to the shepherd, the sheep can eat in peace. As Christians, so can we. The Lord is our Shepherd. How does it reflect on Him when we are sick and tired? He does not look like a Good Shepherd when we are unhealthy and lethargic. Or when we are worried about what we are going to eat or where we are going to find it. Our health status is a marker of how well taken care of we are. Are we close to the Shepherd, or have we wandered off?

In the Gospels, we read the story of when Jesus was in the boat, and the storm was raging. While in the chaos, He simply said, "Peace, be still." Immediately everything calmed down. How often do we find ourselves in a storm of information and conflicting advice? Eat this. Do not eat that. Now you can eat what you were not supposed to eat. Why does the instruction change? Whose best interest are they looking out for? Are they telling the truth or trying to get you to buy their product? Will science ever reach the point where it is not necessary to study the chemical makeup and nutritional benefit of food? Will it ever be unanimously agreed that they know everything they need to know? I highly doubt it. Until that time, differing opinions and conflicting data will abound.

When we focus on which food prevents what sickness, how much we are supposed to eat, and which foods we are supposed to avoid eating, we can get tossed about as well. You try a diet for a short while. It does not work even though the expert or celebrity pitchman guaranteed it would despite the fine print at the bottom of the TV screen. You try eating healthier only to find that the food choices they recommended are now no longer considered healthy. Who has the time or energy to keep up?

Remember, peace is wholeness. Nothing is missing; there are no deficiencies. I believe that includes what our body needs. Peace is the relationship with God. All our needs are provided by the Good Shepherd, who feeds us well. And peace comes from knowing that we will hear what God tells us to eat. John 10:27 guarantees, "My sheep hear My voice."

The Word of God is His voice. We can easily be tossed about, led astray, or frustratingly confused, just like Eve was when we don't know what His Word says. In many places in the Bible, the Lord talks about how He will make sure we have food to eat. Like the birds, He will take care of it. But because we have placed so much emphasis on the healing potential of food, we believe food is all we need, when instead, Jesus's death on the cross took away the diseases and sicknesses.

In John 10:10, He tells us that "I have come that they may have life, and that they may have it more abundantly." The Lord designed eating to be a part of life. Under the care of the Shepherd, there is no lack. When the Israelites were in the Wilderness, God provided manna for them to eat every day. And there wasn't one who was sick during the 40-year wandering.

We must come to a place where we know who we can trust and when we realize that God is the same yesterday, today and forever, His Word is that firm foundation. We don't have to be tossed about with the external influences like the conflicting data and biased advertising. When the food industry uses its methods to persuade you to eat a certain way, cross-check it with what the Health Manual says.

God will never force you to do anything. You must step into the greater understanding and measure of peace that He has already made available for you. Contrary to the steps the world outlines for your health, the Bible's actions are hugely different. His Word is health to all your flesh (Proverbs 4:22). God designed our bodies to function in a predictable way. When we are out of peace or, in other words, in stress or worry, one of the first things that happens is that our digestive system becomes altered or compromised. He knows this is how we function. When people live in this condition 24/7 but still introduce food into a system that is not operating at capacity, there will be physical and mental consequences. When Adam said he was "afraid" in the Garden, his nervous system immediately switched to a fight or flight state. He fled and hid behind a tree. The physical relationship with food changed at that moment.

Philippians 4:6-7 tells us that "the peace of God, which surpasses all understanding, will guard your hearts and minds through Christ Jesus." It's God's peace. It is not that we must try to muster more peace. But we do have to protect it. It's a peace unlike what the world is trying to sell us. He told the disciples, "My peace I leave with you." There's peace, and then there's His peace.

When there is peace, there is no battle or struggle. When there is peace, nothing is lacking. When there is peace, there is wholeness. For most of us, our relationship with food is a constant quest of trial and error. There is a lot of mental energy expended when trying to understand food. The food industry has made it complicated yet deceptively rewarding. It tastes good—really good. It's visually appealing. A ton of marketing and testing has been done to make sure that the message is perfect.

We worry about our food. What's in it? A quick trip to the grocery store can include the unpleasant pop-quiz of questions such as "Is this organic? Has it been sprayed with Roundup? Am I getting all the nutrition I need for the money I'm about to spend?" Just like the world, we have justifiable reasons to worry about food and to lose our peace while we obsess over what to eat. My husband found a cartoon in which Jesus was standing in front of the crowd of 5,000 holding up the loaves and the fish. He was getting ready to give thanks and multiply the food. Someone from the hungry crowd raises their hand and asks, "Are those loaves gluten-free, and do those fish contain high levels of mercury?" That is a humorous and accurate caption of the concerns we have about the quality of our food today.

These conditions we are worried about are man-made. And they are significant causes for concern. But God promises that He will take care of us. He will feed us. If that means avoiding a certain type of food, then you need to do that. Look to the Lord for His guidance with your specific needs. He will enable you to make the choices you need to make. I believe that when we rely on Him, He will provide us with the information we need at the right time. Often, I will notice a food-related topic begins showing up over and over. I have learned to start paying attention. If the Lord is bringing this information to me, then it is time that I know it. I cannot know everything about food. The data is voluminous and always changing. But I can rest in knowing the Creator of the food is also the One who knows what I need. I will protect my peace while the Good Shepherd takes care of all my needs.

Do not worry about what you are going to eat. Why? Because as He promises in Isaiah 55:12, "You will go out in joy and be led forth in peace." Food isn't supposed to make us sad. Remember the Fiber One commercial where the wife hands the husband the box of fiber bars that she wants him to begin eating every day? He takes it, and with a pitiful voice, responds, "Fiber makes me sad." Food is not supposed to make us feel bad. When you are trying to figure out what to do, talk to Him. He will lead you. He won't lead you to eat foods that you hate. It will be with peace and joy, wholeness, and success, all because of your relationship with Him.

I think it is safe to say when a person begins dieting or changing their food in any way, there is little peace. We wonder how much effort is going to be required. We are not convinced we will be able to do it. You hope this will provide the results this time. The Lord promises He will lead us forth in peace and joy. Notice the direction is "forth," but He does not say it will be in a straight, predictable line. When we let the Lord guide us, He will always take us forward. On our own, we often take one step forward and two steps back. We lose the weight then gain it all back and then some. Knowing we are overwhelmed by the mountain, God gives us one step at a time. What is He telling you to do? Is it just to drink more water? We attempt goals, ultimately the opposite way. We tell ourselves, "Ok, I'm going to drink water in ounces based on ½ my body weight. I am going to cut my carbohydrates, AND I'm not going to eat any sugar. I am going to go to the gym eight times a week, AND I am going to wake up an hour earlier every day and workout before I go to work." Where is the peace in that? That is a setup for burnout and failure!

When God guide us, He only shows us one step at a time. Once we take that step, He then shows us the next step. Remember, doing it His way, He leads us "forth" in peace and joy. Peace and joy come from a personal sense of accomplishment. Instead of feeling like a repeated failure with an insufficient amount of willpower, we can competently and successfully take one step at a time. Do you feel joyous when you accomplish a goal? Do you feel happy when you begin to see yourself as a success? That has been the Lord's plan for you all along. In Joshua 1:8, He promises that you will have "good success."

The complexity and confusion of food is not an environment that fosters peace. How do you know if you are eating enough or too much? Or is what you are eating the wrong food for you? Stress and anxiety can get overwhelming. If you do not get your food right, the consequences can be fatal. With God's peace, you can rest. You have a Guide who knows what you need. He has the plan designed for you and you alone. It can be as simple as adding one thing to your diet; then next, you feel prompted to remove one thing from your diet. The beauty is that only you and God know. He has a peace that you will not find anywhere else, including food.

He wants you to be successful. In Proverbs 16:3, we read, "Commit to the Lord whatever you do, and he will establish your plans."

Stop looking for the next diet to try. Stop listening to what all the "experts" are saying you need to eat or avoid eating. Instead, the missing ingredient to your food and diet success has been God. In Psalm 37:4, we are told to "Take delight in the Lord, and he will give you the desires of your heart." He said, "desires." Not needs. Religious Christians believe that God is only interested in meeting our needs. We should not ask for our wants. Doing so is too indulgent. What do you desire when it comes to food? He is inviting you into a relationship with Him in which there is no off-limit topics. Yes, He is keeping the universe in place. He is listening to and answering everyone's prayers. But what you eat matters to Him all the same. Imagine how happy He will be if every time you think about food or are getting ready to eat, you talk to Him about it. Will you make mistakes? Absolutely! But He is bigger than those. He can even correct it.

Proverbs 3:5-6 "Trust in the Lord with all your heart and lean not on your own understanding; in all your ways submit to him, and he will make your paths straight."

Let go of the way our culture typically sees food. Instead, focus on the food-Giver who has also promised to give you His peace. You will know the direction you are supposed to go and the choices that you are supposed to make. With God, it will not be an overwhelming task. And you have a guarantee of success. His peace will guide you. If you do not feel peaceful about incorporating seaweed into your diet, then don't do it. If drinking one glass of water in place of one of the soft drinks you typically consume every day makes you comfortable, then that is what you do. The guarantee of success occurs because He has shown you the next step to take. He is leading you forth in peace and joy. He has also provided you with a special anointing to accomplish it. All you need to do is take the step. That is a much better approach than a diet, don't you think?

CHAPTER 9

WISDOM

When I graduated with my master's degree, I experienced a variety of emotions. I was thrilled that it was over. I felt a strong sense of accomplishment, having finished a 2-year program in 1 ½ years, but I was tired. My brain was tired. Yet, I was excited about all the new nutritional knowledge and understanding I had acquired. I was also slightly disappointed by the fact that, even after earning the degree, I could not definitively say I understood all the complexities of food. Don't get me wrong; I learned a lot. I loved the program. Due to the ever-changing perspectives about food, I realized that learning could never be complete. There's virtually no way to know everything there is to know about food. Apart from that, not everyone has the time, the resources, or even the interest in understanding food at an advanced-degree level. Thankfully, the Lord never intended for food to be so complicated.

I think it has become so because we have attached many health consequences to it, and we are looking at food from only an intellectual perspective. God created us with a body, soul, and spirit. With the body, we interact with the world around us, in other words, the physical world. Our soul is comprised of our appetites, desires, and senses. The spirit part helps us connect with and relate to God. All three are equally important.

For the Christian, we must understand food in connection with the three parts of man. People tend to associate food with the body and the soul. For example, we are motivated to make food decisions based on how our diet has affected the body. Or, on the other hand, how we want our body to respond. If we are overweight, we consider changing our food. If we are sick, we seek food that will make us well again. From the soul perspective, we make food decisions based on our appetite and desire. Bringing the forkful of moist, chocolate cake to our mouth, we are not considering whether it will spend "a moment on the lips and a lifetime on the hips."

Learning about nutrition requires research, study, data, and knowledge. These intellectual pursuits fall into the soul realm of man. How food relates to the spirit is typically overlooked. Without the spiritual for us, only ⅔ of the man is considered. Remember, we talked about how acquiring more food knowledge has left many of us more confused? It's because we are only focused on the soul. We need the full picture. To understand food's relationship to the spirit, we can consult God's Word. The Bible is spirit. It was written by inspiration from God, and it addresses the topic of food.

We are instructed to eat our veggies and to stay away from red meat. At the time of this writing, we are encouraged to avoid carbohydrates. Based on repeated historical experience, we all know that given enough time, that advice is likely to change.

Instead of the Lord expecting everyone to acquire a level of food knowledge, He instead has given us the gift of wisdom. Years ago, I heard a pastor teach that wisdom means knowing what to do when you don't know what to do. Can anyone relate to that feeling? How about when you are staring at the menu of your favorite restaurant? How do you decide the best option among all those meal choices? They give you a description of what each entrée includes, but they don't tell you about the oil in which the vegetables are sautéed. Nor do they tell you what type of butter they provided for your baked potato. Is it butter real, or is it a vegetable oil spread? In a reversal of advice, butter is now considered healthy, while vegetable oil is not.

Furthermore, I dare say, you don't know how clean the kitchen is or the hands that plated your food or carried your plate to the table. How about when you are in the grocery store trying to run in and run out quickly? When grocery shopping is just another chore on your list of things to do, the last thing you have time for is to read all the labels and compare healthy options. Whenever I go to the grocery store, walking toward the store entrance, I ask the Lord for wisdom. I invite Him to guide me in selecting what I need and to avoid what I don't. There have been times after leaving the store that I remember something I had intended to buy. Then I remember that I had asked the Lord for guidance. For whatever reason, He didn't bring it to mind while I was in the store. The item wasn't for me to purchase during that shopping trip.

Grocery shopping is especially complicated when you do it hungry. Perhaps complicated is not the word. Maybe it is more of a lost cause. Everything looks delicious, quick, and convenient. All diet- related reasoning goes out of the window. So, in those instances, let the Lord shop with you. If you get a prompting to eat a snack before you shop, then do it. The Lord is preparing you to make wise decisions. If there is something on your list that you just do not feel that you are supposed to purchase, then don't do it. The Lord is directing your decisions.

Do not go into the grocery store on autopilot. A vast amount of marketing research has been conducted, expecting and catering to zombie-like shoppers. When you are vulnerable, the industry hopes to entice you to purchase what you do not necessarily need and that which is most likely contrary to your goals. We get into a rut of buying the same foods out of habit. We know the exact location on the shelf. The grocery store knows this too. There is a science to the placement of food on a store shelf. The Bull's Eye Zone is comprised of the second and third shelves from the top. This zone is where the most expensive foods are placed. The food manufacturers must pay premium prices for their items to reside there. Considering that shoppers tend to purchase items that are eye level, it makes financial sense for the manufacturer to want their product as visible as possible.[1]

Considering all the science and manipulative advertising tactics waiting for you when you walk into your local grocery store, the consumer needs reinforcement. Often, the shopping is unplanned, last-minute, and the least enjoyable chore on the day's to-do list. Entering this maze of food mind games when you are tired, weak, or hungry is a recipe for spending more money than you planned or getting more convenient processed foods than you had intended.

The grocery store can be a unique place to talk to Him. Think about it. Along the periphery of the store, you are surrounded by a variety of the foods He created. The grocery store is an intersection of His food and man's food packaged in a creative way to get you to buy more. Slow down a bit and take it all in. Listen for His direction. Ask Him questions. It is a time to interact with the Creator. Picture it. Look at the colors, the provision, and the variety just in the produce department alone. He knows you need it, and He also knows precisely what you and your family need nutritionally.

People routinely state that feeding themselves and their family healthier options is too expensive. It is cheaper to buy highly processed, nutritionally void, and calorie-dense foods. However, maybe it is not as expensive as we've been led to believe. In a December 5, 2013 BMJ (British Medical Journal) Open article, a study was published in which "The researchers found that healthier diet patterns — for example, diets rich in fruits, vegetables, fish, and nuts — cost significantly more than unhealthy diets (for example, those rich in processed foods, meats, and refined grains). On average, a day's worth of the healthiest diet patterns cost about $1.50

more per day than the least healthy ones." I thought it would have been a lot more than $1.50.

The article further reports "The researchers suggested that unhealthy diets may cost less because food policies have focused on the production of "inexpensive, high volume" commodities, which have led to "a complex network of farming, storage, transportation, processing, manufacturing, and marketing capabilities that favor sales of highly processed food products for maximal industry profit."

I get it; there is nothing worse than buying that bag of organic kale only to throw it out a month later. I know. It got lost in the crisper drawer — wink, wink. The now-liquid contents are only identifiable by the label on the front of the bag, reminding you that, in its heyday, it was kale. No one wants to waste money. The Lord does not want you to waste your money either. If you ask Him for wisdom, and He does not direct you to buy kale, then don't buy it. Even if the Internet is telling you that kale is all the rage and that it is the new potato chip, do not buy it. Trust in the wisdom He is giving you. It is your wisdom for that moment for you and your family.

The Bible tells us that He wants us to ask for wisdom and then ask for even more. He provides us with abundant wisdom. And He does it without finding fault. I do not believe that the Lord expects us to obsess over what vitamins are in which foods unless that's something you get excited over. He simply wants our food to be an invitation to talk to Him and to include Him in our day-to-day decisions, even when going to the grocery store is the chore most people dislike doing.

Daily we are bombarded with messages regarding diet and weight loss programs. The advertisements are on television, in magazines, doctor's offices and the Internet. There is a constant focus on changing what and how much you eat for you to lose weight and feel better. That is not to say that people do not need to lose weight. It is probably the most declared New Year's resolution every year. January 1 rolls around, and people take off with gusto on this new quest to lose weight. And it is legitimate. They honestly hope this time they can be successful. It is easy to make that promise to yourself around the first of every year because, let's face it, we all have relaxed our eating standards during the holidays. Has anyone ever thought it unfair that Halloween, Thanksgiving, and Christmas are within the last three months of the year? Such scheduling creates a lot of work for January. Though I do not have science or data to support my theory, I feel certain that more calories are consumed on those days than any other day of the year. We know those days are coming, and we give ourselves permission to indulge and enjoy with the stipulation that we will change on January 1st. According to Inc.com, "Studies show that about 60% of us make New Year's resolutions each year. Sadly, only about 8% achieve them."[2]

The book of Proverbs in the Old Testament is considered the Book of Wisdom. To paraphrase Dave Ramsey, reading Proverbs every day provides wisdom equivalent to getting a master's degree. When you operate in wisdom, it is much better and more effective than book smarts. God's wisdom doesn't just apply to one area of your life. It covers every area. Remember, relying on your knowledge impacts your soul. Reading God's Word feeds your spirit.

One of the ways we know how vital wisdom is to our daily lives is the quantity in which God is willing to provide it to us. James 1:5 tells us, "If any of you lacks wisdom, you should ask God, who gives generously to all without finding fault, and it will be given to you." The verse continues with one condition, "But when you ask, you must believe and not doubt." When you are asking for wisdom regarding your relationship with food, the Lord has promised that you will have it. The only requirement is that we must ask. In our daily life, there are countless opportunities for us to ask for His wisdom regarding food. We can ask for wisdom for our meals, our grocery shopping, as well as what foods to include and exclude from our diet. We can walk in wisdom no matter what or where we are. Knowing that He has promised to provide generously, we can expect to make wise decisions when we include Him. The solution to any challenge or problem we face is the wisdom of God. Wisdom will help you know what to eat and what to avoid.

Years ago, when my husband was interested in losing some weight, he tried all the fad diets of the time. They were either too restrictive or too difficult to fit into his lifestyle. The constant cycle of yet another failed diet is one of the consequences of tackling a food issue on your own. Dieting is hard. It is a physical and emotional stress on your body. And not all diets are for everyone. The word "diet" in Greek means "lifestyle." Our culture devises diets that can be so extreme there is no way it can be successfully implemented long term. The severe caloric restriction is just too dangerous, or the limited food options are just too dull. So instead, my husband decided to take His Father at His Word. He asked the Lord for wisdom. He specifically wanted wisdom to know how to feed his body and adopt a way of eating that can last a lifetime. They came up with a successful "lifestyle" for him. Now, this diet will not likely work if I tried it because the Lord designed it for my husband. My husband asked for wisdom and believed that he received it because the Lord promised to supply it generously. With the Lord's wisdom at the forefront of his mind, my husband feels confident regarding any food decision made. The Lord created each one of us, unique from each other. We have different talents and abilities. We look different. We even come from different places in this world. Weston Price, a Canadian dentist, found that, based on the area, the inhabitants ate a diet unique to them. The collective information showed that some groups lived successfully and healthfully off a high percentage fat diet; others did well consuming meat. Other groups had a more balanced diet among vegetables, meat, and fat. The point is one diet is not suitable for everyone.

I attended a conference during which Dr. Nicholas Gonzalez presented his research regarding nutrition and cancer. He talked about the work of a mentor, Dr. Kelley, who cured himself of cancer by eating a vegetarian diet. His form of cancer caused visible tumors on his abdomen. When he ate non-vegetarian foods, the tumors visibly grew. When he ate vegetarian, he could see the tumors shrink. Following his body's response to food, Dr. Kelley made a full recovery. Years later, his wife developed cancer. Knowing the diet worked for him, he fed her the same vegetarian diet. With every meal, she became increasingly sicker. Against his better judgment and out of fear that without making a change, she would die, he began feeding her red meat. To his surprise, she responded so favorably that he fed her red meat for every meal. She eventually made a full recovery. Based on his personal life and death research, he realized that every person needs a different diet.

Our bodies and our nutritional needs are different. So how could one diet work for every person? Everyone reacts differently to food. Everyone has different tastes. One of the most significant challenges and contributing factors to the failure of many diets is that typically people don't like the food they are limited to eating. How are you supposed to stick to limited food options when you don't enjoy the food on the menu? The simple answer is you cannot. Diets tend to be a short-term fix with long-term consequences such as altered metabolism, regaining all the weight, and not wanting to try dieting ever again.

The lure of wisdom is seen in Genesis 3:6 "When the woman saw that the fruit of the tree was good for food and pleasing to the eye, and also desirable for gaining wisdom, she took some and ate it." Now up to this point, the association of wisdom with food was never established. God never told her that wisdom could be attained from her diet. We read in Proverbs 2:6, "For the Lord gives wisdom." If Adam and Eve needed wisdom in the Garden, He would have given it to them. In 1 Kings 4:29-30, "God gave Solomon wisdom and understanding beyond measure ... so that Solomon's wisdom surpassed the wisdom of all the people of the east and all the wisdom of Egypt." In verse 33, we read that in Solomon's wisdom, he spoke about plant life and animals. He spoke about food. Solomon is reputed to be the wisest man ever to live. Notice that Solomon asked for wisdom. Confident in his relationship with the Lord, he could have asked for anything. But he asked for wisdom, which pleased the Lord.

Today it seems that to feed ourselves in the healthiest way possible, we need to know a lot of detail and information about food. We need to know what to eat, when to eat it, and how much to eat. Instead of making our nourishment decisions based on the ever-changing knowledge of science and authority, as Christians, we have something even better. We have God's wisdom. Wisdom is always better than knowledge.

There is practical wisdom in God's Word related to our food. Studying nutrition can be complicated. There are numerous ways of eating, depending upon the person. One person can have diabetes; another could be battling cancer, while a third wants to lose weight. Each person requires a different diet composition and eating schedule. Being the Creator of your body, God knows what you need. Have you ever been in a situation in which you find that you keep hearing about a specific food? For example, without seeking it out, you keep hearing about how you should avoid sugar. Or how you should only eat two times a day. When you get these indications, ask the Lord if He is providing you with wisdom in how to fuel your body correctly.

In Ephesians 1:17, the Scripture tells us the apostle Paul is asking "that the God of our Lord Jesus Christ, the Father of glory, may give to you the spirit of wisdom."

In Proverbs 4:7, we read that "wisdom is the principal thing; therefore get wisdom." That's pretty clear. Often, we think that wisdom is necessary for only the big decisions or choices in life. And it is. It's also available for every small decision or choice we must make. God didn't outline limitations for which we can ask for wisdom. But considering the importance of feeding our bodies and navigating through the labyrinth of misinformation and financial gain, there's never been a time more needing of wisdom. And as Christians, we have access to all the wisdom we need. We just need to ask.

Having wisdom has nothing to do with education. It has nothing to do with how much knowledge you have acquired about food. Remember, wisdom is knowing what to do when you don't know what to do. Wisdom is spiritual. For lack of a better explanation, wisdom is a "knowing." It's a confidence that the decisions you make are right for you. Someone else's wisdom may look completely different, and that's okay. Your wisdom is between you and the wisdom-Giver.

Part of the wisdom is knowing God's perspective about food and what His Word already tells us. Feed on His Word. When you do this, you are acquiring wisdom. When you are reading the Scripture, pay attention to what He is speaking to your heart. Remember, those who seek Him find Him. He is not going to make it complicated. Instead, He has given us wisdom so that we can enjoy and get the benefit of the food He created.

As I have said, the book of Proverbs is the Book of Wisdom. In a couple of places, God discusses food. In Proverbs 9:5, Wisdom provides us with the invitation to "Come, eat my food." We do not have to search for wisdom. It's not in a textbook. We just need to tune our ear to wisdom's voice. Wisdom is inviting you to fellowship with her. Her food is what your body needs. The invitation stands, and all you must to do is accept it. If wisdom is guiding you, then there's no reason to worry if the food will taste good or be right for you. Nowadays, we especially need wisdom amidst all the confusion. The food industry is skillfully trying to persuade us to buy their food. It is their job to make a profit. The more we eat it, the more they make and sell to us. The food industry uses cravings and addictions to keep us wanting and coming back for more. Often, we don't have enough knowledge to protect ourselves. But with wisdom, we do.

Wisdom's entire focus is for our benefit. God provides wisdom with no expectation of anything in return. In Proverbs 9:6, Wisdom invites us to "Come ... leave the company of the ignorant people, and live." The term "ignorant" is not an insult. It is describing those individuals that don't know wisdom is available. They are seeking after knowledge alone. As fast as knowledge is changing, it will never be enough.

How often do you ask yourself, "What should I eat?" Several voices are trying to influence that vitally important decision. Take a moment to ask for wisdom. The Lord knows your body better than you do, and significantly more than the food industry does. When you ask for wisdom, He will direct you to what He knows you need at that very moment. Isn't that wonderful? What a relief! It was never the Lord's plan for us to struggle under the weight of confusion and guilt surrounding food. Instead, He has given us an answer, and it is found in wisdom. If He knows the number of hairs on your head, considering that He has taken the time to count them, then how you feed yourself is infinitely more important, and it matters to Him. He wants to guide you with a generous supply of wisdom.

In the Book of Wisdom, Proverbs 30:8 says, "So give me only as much food as I need." Wow! Did anyone else feel their toes crunch? It is so hard to stop eating when the food tastes good! Research shows that it takes about 20 minutes for the brain to register that the body is full. Time must be allowed for the hormones of satiety or fullness to reach the brain. Fortunately, we don't live in a perpetual state of hunger. That would be awful. In a healthy body, the hormones are there to do their job and tell you it's time to put the fork down.

In our super-sized, 24-hour 7-day a week access, food-obsessed culture, this verse is quite relevant. People are consumed with how much they should eat. How many calories? How much protein? There's no denying that we need food. Our bodies need food in the right amounts, and when it is provided too much, the body knows how to handle it. We just don't like the consequences: upset stomach, bloated feeling, or, over the long-term, fat accumulation. Initially, it was believed that the body immediately began storing excess calories. But recently, it has been shown that in most instances, the body increases its energy output to accommodate the occasional caloric increase. The body is well-equipped to store the excess for a rainy day. Sadly, by the looks of many Americans, we must be predicting a lot of rain. Health consequences are occurring at a rapid rate. The medical industry will tell you that the root of the issue is that people simply overeat. But then you have the food industry more than willing to help you consume as much as you want.

There are a lot of factors that must be considered, such as activity level, health state, fitness goals, pregnancy, and others. There is no "one size fits all" intake level. My husband is 6'2". I am 5'5". The amount of food on our dinner plates should not really look the same. If they do, one of us is eating too much or not enough. So how do you know which one it is?

It is not by coincidence that food marketers advertise, "no one can eat just one." Am I referring to carrots? I think not. I bet you have already pictured the salty, potato-y snack I'm talking about here. We are working against a marketing plan that has scientifically and methodically manipulated the food so that your brain continues to crave more. The resulting food-like substances provide little to no nutritional value with empty calories and unhealthy chemicals.

On the other hand, the food the Lord provides is satisfying and satiating. Once the body is satisfied with real food, you do not need or want to eat additional food beyond your body's needs. The Lord's food is loaded with healthy nutrients and calories that your body is designed to use efficiently and effectively.

Praying "Give me only as much food as I need" is the secret weapon in the fight against overeating. This is His wisdom. You are just taking Him at His Word. You have the successful interplay between the soul's appetite, the body's needs, and the spiritual guidance. I believe that this is a state of complete nourishment.

Your body recognizes and knows what to do with real food. Unfortunately, the body is not designed to routinely compensate for the nutritionally void, calorically dense items we shove in our mouth. For example, when we eat real foods that have not been cooked, our body responds favorably. However, when we ingest foods that have been cooked or processed, we experience something called "digestive leukocytosis." The body's immune system mobilizes the white blood cells to deal with the stress of the altered food. If we ingest highly processed foods, studies show the "digestive leukocytosis" is at a level akin to the white blood cell mobilization when a virus or a bacteria has invaded the body. From start to finish, the process takes about 90 minutes.

In Proverbs 24:13, we are told, "My son, eat honey because it is good." In our culture today, anything sweet is looked upon with healthy skepticism. You know you want it, but it is not good for you. Here the Lord is telling us, despite what culture is directing us to do, anything He made is good to eat. Here is a loving Father telling His son, "Eat it, and enjoy it. I made it for you. I know it's good."

This is how to use wisdom in our food choices. First, if

God made it, then eat it. Then, ask Him to direct you regarding how much food you need at that meal or throughout the day. He designed your body to need food to function well. Many believe that the Lord is too busy to be troubled with what they eat every day; it is insignificant to Him. In John 4:32, He told the disciples, "I have food to eat of which you do not know." When we talk to Him about our food, it feeds Him. He craves your communication. He wants to give you the wisdom to make the right choices for you and your family. He is just waiting for you to ask. He wants you to get the most significant benefit of what you eat. Then when you do eat it, enjoy it.

CHAPTER 10

THANKSGIVING

In John 16:23, we read the promise, "Most assuredly, I say to you, whatever you ask the Father in My name He will give you." This is a verse that most Christians are generally familiar with. However, Christians who believe this verse are criticized by non-Christians and Christians alike. They are accused of believing in a "prosperity theology." Those who do not believe in prosperity will say, "You can't ask for a million dollars in Jesus's name." Or, from a non-financial perspective, "At 5'6" you can't ask to become 6 feet tall in Jesus's name." As with anything, you can take it to the extreme. Truthfully, Jesus's name is not a magic wand. But there is something incredibly powerful about it. If you are asking for things in Jesus's name that God has already promised are yours, then you are merely coming into agreement with God the Father. You are acknowledging that you are not asking in your stead, but rather, you can make the request because of His precious Son, Jesus.

Anytime you remind God of His Son, Jesus, you make Him smile, and He responds as promised.

For the Christian, this is important to know. When the verse tells us that we can ask for "whatever," I want to know what "whatever" means. If I am guaranteed "whatever" when I ask in Jesus's name, I would like to have it, whatever it is. According to the Strongest NIV Exhaustive Concordance, the term "whatever" in the Greek language is "tis," which means "anything" or "whatever." Often, this verse is taught in the context of finances, health, or things we need in our daily living. Shouldn't food fall into that category as well? What do you want in connection with your food? Have you ever thought about that?

We have been permitted to ask for things in Jesus's name, and we can do this daily when praying over our food before we consume it. In Psalms 23:1, we read, "The Lord is my shepherd, I lack nothing." If you have the faith to believe that He will give you whatever you ask in His name, then, when coming into agreement with Him, shouldn't your food always be precisely what you need? Most families have their tradition of praying over their meal. It typically includes a memorized prayer most likely handed down from previous generations. In my family, the prayer goes something like this: "Father in Heaven, thank you for this food that you have provided for us. We ask that you nourish our bodies to Your goodness, in Jesus's name. Amen." Taking Jesus's promise of

John 16:23 at His Word, my "whatever" is that our bodies be nourished by the food we are about to eat. "In Jesus's name" is the "whatever activator." He then nourishes our bodies to His ability, not the food's ability. When you break it down, it's not complicated. Imagine what it does to God's heart when He hears a little one learning that they, too, can thank Jesus for the food and ask that it nourish their body.

Now, let's take it one step further. In Ephesians 3:20, God tells us He is "able to do immeasurably more than all we can ask or imagine, according to His power that is at work within us." Let me get this straight. For our purposes here, we can ask for "whatever" in connection with our food, and He will give it to us. Then, after we ask, He can do even more than we ask or imagine. And not only more, but the "more" is incapable of being measured. We tend to measure our nutrition by grams, calories, and percentages. Some people count calories. Others focus on consuming a certain gram number of macronutrients a day. Food labels are written so you can readily see the percentage of the daily value that a food item will provide you. Nutrition is measured. God can do immeasurably more. Maybe it's because I am not particularly good at math, and that's putting it mildly, but knowing that He can provide exponentially more benefit than what I can calculate is a good feeling.

When we pray over our meal, we are following Jesus's actions. In all four of the gospels, we read the personalized account of Jesus feeding the 5,000 people who had come to hear Him preach on the mountain. Knowing that the attendees were hungry, Jesus accepted the five loaves and two fish from a little boy. For that many people, the tiny lunch was woefully inadequate to feed and meet every nutritional need. Completely unphased by the paltry amount, Jesus simply thanked His Father for the provision. At that moment, though not visible to onlookers, the physical amount of the food miraculously changed. It multiplied! So much so that everyone present was able to eat until satisfied. There were even twelve baskets of food leftover. Following Jesus's example, can you see the power of thanking the Father for the provision of your food? This instance wasn't the only time this occurred. Not only did He feed the 5,000 people on the mountain that day, but He also performed the same miracle for 4,000 additional people on another occasion. From a nutritional standpoint, you can't tell me that 9,000 people all had the same dietary need or requirements. Yet He met each one... easily.

The disciples had a different focus. When Jesus instructed them to find food to feed the hungry crowd, the disciples recognized the impossibility of the task. In John 6:7, Philip answered Jesus, "It would take more than half a year's wages to buy enough bread for each one to have a bite!" The disciples could only see the insufficiency. There's no mention of them even discussing the nutritional needs. The cost was their primary focus. Often this is the primary focus for many families. Find cheaper food at higher quantities with little to no thought of the nutritional value.

In the disciples' wildest dreams, an ordinary lunch of

bread and fish would never be good enough to feed all those hungry mouths. I've heard it preached that the number 5,000 only accounted for the men. The women and children were not included. For our purposes here, let's go with that. According to a statistic by Gretchen Livingston, in 2015, women have "2. 4 children on average."[1]

Just for kicks and giggles, doing the math, by today's standards, that's 5,000 men; 5,000 women, and 12,000 kids. That's 22,000 people to feed with an ordinary brown bag lunch. And Jesus accomplished it by thanking God for the provision. Amazing!

The Bible does not mention the nutritional value of the food that was consumed on either the 5,000 or 4,000-person occasion. I believe that omission is intentional. If the focus were on the protein, carbohydrate, and fats, it would have become too complicated. Furthermore, with Jesus, that information did not matter. It was irrelevant to His ability to be able to feed and nourish more than adequately every person attending.

Simply put, He took the ordinary lunch of a small boy and performed a nutritional miracle. Just like He promises for us in Ephesians, He did more than the disciples could have asked or imagined. In Jesus's hands, the composition and quantity of the food changed. Notice the route the brown bag meal took. The boy's mother presumably prepared his ordinary lunch for the day, providing him with just enough to support his activity. Recognizing the need for a larger group of people, the boy still brought all he had to Jesus. He did not give the food to the disciples who were preoccupied with the financial distractions. Just like today, when we are ready to eat the ordinary meal prepared by our hands or those of another person, and we allow Jesus to be part of it, it becomes exactly what we need.

When we say a prayer of thanks for our food, we are talking to the same Father Jesus did. So, why should the impact on our diet not be any different? Jesus expected it to multiply. Jesus expected His need for more food to be met. He believed that His Father would also meet the nutritional needs of everyone present. Jesus did not take the boy's lunch, then go off by Himself and talk to His Father for 30 minutes about what needed to be done or changed for the food to get the most significant impact. He simply thanked His Father for the provision. Shouldn't we at least be able to believe that He is interested enough in our meal to specifically meet the nutritional needs of each person around our table? At our table, we typically are surrounded by loved ones, people whose presence and health matter to us. We want their nutritional needs met. We do not want them to struggle. Someone has taken the time to prepare the food to gather together. What a precious time for fellowship and nourishment! With Jesus, the nourishment is exponential and individually targeted.

In our hectic, drive-thru, eat behind the wheel, day to day living, we are in such a rush that we fail to take the time to do the most essential thing: to pray over the food. Are we always going to make the perfect meal? No. Are we always going to make the right choice? No. Jesus is not only going to bless the food if it is organic, non-genetically modified, and cooked in cast iron. He did not criticize the little boy for sharing His food when it was obviously insufficient. We don't read anywhere in the four gospel accounts that Jesus ever asked the child, "How am I supposed to work with this? This is not good enough. Do you know how many people on this mountain can't eat gluten?!" Nope. Jesus operates best with the insufficient and the ordinary. This little boy probably did not even plan his meal, and what he carried in that small brown bag was likely packaged because it was all his mother had to give him. But in Jesus's hands, it became what everyone else needed.

I think it is interesting that there's no mention of the boy beyond the donation of the food. Letting my imagination wander a bit, I can imagine him sitting right beside Jesus while they ate together. I can see Jesus putting His arm around the boy and loving Him. I can picture his little chest poked out because Jesus performed a miracle with his lunch. That boy's life was forever changed by that very moment. Witnessing the miracle, I'm sure he never doubted what Jesus could do. Maybe it's not mentioned in the Bible because it was a private conversation or exchange between Jesus and a boy who was willing to share his ordinary brown bag lunch. Seeing the disciples frantically collecting and counting the coins from their tunic pockets, the little boy could have thought to himself, "I sure wish I could help, but I definitely don't have enough to feed everybody," and then he walks away. The boy showed Jesus his measure of faith. "This is all I have, but I know you can do something amazing with it."

Just like this little guy, be willing to share your food with Jesus. Do like He did and thank the Father for its provision. Have faith that it matters to Jesus, and He knows what your body needs at that moment. He did it for thousands at one time. He can do it for you and the loved ones gathered around your table. Not only can He do it, more importantly, He will do it.

In Genesis 17, God is referred to as El Shaddai. The names of God have always been fascinating to me, especially Jehovah Rapha, the Healer. The names reflect an aspect of God. El Shaddai has been taught to mean God Almighty. While this is true, according to the Scofield Bible Study tools, El Shaddai also has an interpretation that is significant to our understanding in this book. "The qualifying word 'Shaddai' is formed from the Hebrew word 'shad,' the breast, invariably used in Scripture for a woman's breast. 'Shaddai,' therefore, means primarily 'the breasted.' God is 'Shaddai,' because He is the Nourisher, the Strength-giver, and so, in a secondary sense, the Satisfier ... so El Shaddai is that name of God which sets Him forth as the Strength-giver and Satisfier of His people. It is on every account to be regretted that 'Shaddai' was translated 'Almighty.' The primary name El or Elohim sufficiently signifies almightiness. 'All-sufficient' would far better express both the Hebrew meaning and the characteristic use of the name in Scripture."

Did you see that? His name means Nourisher! Because it's who He is, it matters to Him that we are fed. Our food is important. A mother knows how to feed her baby. Her body produces what her precious child needs to become strong and healthy. Yet while the mother doesn't nurse the child forever, the name El Shaddai teaches us that God will. We never age out of His interest in or ability to nourishing us. No matter our age, no matter the need, He is as focused as a new mother on making sure that we are fed. To wear the title "Nourisher," we must need nourishing. It's the nature of the relationship. Isn't that beautiful?

He knows what we need. We just need to ask. A baby will ask its mother for food by crying. It lets momma know it's hungry. Talk to Him about your diet. Ask Him to show you how best to nourish your body. The One who created it would surely know best, don't you think? It is so important to Him that He called Himself El Shaddai.

Here in the south, when we gather around the table, someone will invariably ask, "Who's going to say the blessing?" or "Who is going to say grace?" Proverbs 18:21 tells us the "The tongue has the power of life and death." In James 3:10, we read that "Out of the same mouth come blessings and curses," which teaches us that there are no neutral words. We are either blessing or cursing, building, or tearing down. In God's economy or His way of successful living, we read in Deuteronomy 30:19 "I have set before you life and death, the blessing and the curse." Do you speak over your food? Do you say a blessing over your food?

Galatians 3:13 teaches us, "Christ redeemed us from the curse of the law by becoming a curse for us, for it is written: 'Cursed is everyone who is hung on a tree.'" Because of the great exchange at the cross, we are supposed to live blessed. When we speak those blessings over the food, the power of life infuses it. Speaking those blessings is a hard concept to grasp for some. But living a different life means making different choices or allowing your perspective to change. The Bible tells us in Romans 12:2 to "be transformed by the renewing of your mind." We can do this by taking a stand on what the Word of God says and how it directs us to live a successful life. The Bible demonstrates that, in Jesus's name, our food can transform into exactly what He knows we need. All we must do is ask Him for "whatever," thank Him for it and have faith that He will do what He has promised. When we say grace or the blessing over the food, we tend to only focus on thanking the Lord for His provision. We've been taught that thanking Him is the right thing to do; we're saying the blessing for His benefit. He deserves our thanks. But there is so much more to it.

It is a foregone conclusion that we can grow food. During the spring and summers, we visit farmer's markets, and the grocery stores advertise "locally-grown" foods. We know a farmer supplied what we are purchasing. Yet, we give little thought to the fact that the Lord commanded the earth to produce the food. When Adam sinned, as part of the punishment, the Lord could have told the earth to stop producing altogether. What a nutritional mess we would be in if that had happened. Thank goodness for His grace! Because of Adam's sin, the ground was cursed. Adam would have to learn to plant and harvest. By not having the Farmer's Almanac Garden of Eden edition, it made growing food a bit more of a challenge. Seeing the Lord's grace when it comes to our food provides an even greater reason to give thanks.

Jesus's death on the cross changed everything for our benefit. The traditional salvation message typically preached from the pulpits every Sunday morning across this country is about salvation from eternal damnation. But salvation is also about health. It includes the food on your plate. So next time you sit down at the table ready to partake of a meal, take a moment to say "grace" or "the blessing." Not out of habit, but instead, knowing that you are talking to your Father, who knows what the food needs to accomplish. Thank the Lord for His provision, for His grace, and His kindness.

When you thank the Lord for the food on your plate, the Lord multiplies the benefits, just like He did with the people on the mountain. And just like the little boy did physically, we can spiritually give back to Him what He created for our consumption. In His hands, the food you and your family will consume while enjoying each other's company will satisfy your body and will meet all the needs. The person who is praying does not have to be formal with all the "thee's" and "thou's." A simple thank you from the heart, as Jesus said to His Father, was more than enough. It will be for you too.

Your words have power. We know this because Psalm 107:2 instruct us, "Let the redeemed of the Lord say so," and Romans 10:6 states, "The righteousness of faith speaks."

Remember, God said, "whatever you ask in My name ..." He did not say, "whatever you think about" or "whatever you wish for." No. He clearly said, "ask." When the family bows their head to say the blessing, someone is speaking aloud talking to the Lord. Imagine what it would be like if the prayer silently prayed to himself on behalf of everyone's food.

There would be a lot of one-eyed room scans for the signal that the prayer was over. There's power in speaking. You have the privilege to use your voice, or better yet, your tongue to speak blessings over the food.

Typically, when it comes to our mouth, the focus is on what goes in it. We are aware of our taste buds. They tend to dictate our food choices. Because of the significance of this one-way traffic pattern, we have neglected the most impactful and health-consequential direction: what comes out of our mouth. Matthew 15:11, tells us "Not that which goeth into the mouth defileth a man; but that which cometh out of the mouth, this defileth a man." Imagine that. What if we have been preoccupied or focused on the wrong direction? Have we been traveling down a one-way street the wrong way? Mark 11:24 tells us, "whatever you ask for in prayer, believe that you have received it, and it will be yours." How often do you make a meal choice only to question, is this enough, or is this the right food for me? It seems like eating for health is just a game of chance. We oftentimes hear of someone falling sick, and friends and family will comment, "But he was so healthy and ate all the right foods!" So why did he still get sick? It feels like we have no control over it. It is just the luck of the draw. But for the Christian, we do have control. We can open our mouth and declare God's Word. What are you saying? What are you asking for in prayer over your food? Do you believe that you will receive it? Through Mark's writing, God promises that "whatever" will be yours.

As Christians, we are children of the Most High God, the King of Kings. That makes us royalty. In Psalm 8:5 we are told that we are "crowned with glory and honor." First Peter 2:9 tells us, "But you are a chosen people, a royal priesthood, a holy nation, God's special possession."

Throughout the Bible, we read of instances where a person was healed from a disease or sickness. In the Old Testament, for it to be official, they would have to present themselves before the priest. Whatever the priest declared was final. In Revelation 5:10, the Bible tells us that the blood of Jesus has "made us kings and priests to our God; And we shall reign on the earth." Each Christian, therefore, is both a king and a priest. In other words, a "royal priest." The authority that comes with this blood-bought position is immense. Just like the priests in Bible times, whatever you declare is final. Furthermore, whatever a king says becomes law. Think of the power you possess to be able to speak over your food. What are you declaring? Nothing?

Are the moments before eating full of your vocal silence? Are the only sounds at the table coming from your fork clanking against your plate? Each time you sit down to eat, there is a powerful moment that most people regrettably lose. They fail to take advantage of the privilege of speaking over their food. What you speak should be based on what you know and what God has already said about your food. Speak with the authority of a royal priest. In faith, believe that what you say is true.

The Lord is telling us to open our mouths. Not just to cram food into it. But to speak. We are to pray over our food with confidence and authority that we are partnering with God to nourish our bodies." Whatever you ask for in Jesus's name, I will give you." Seems straightforward. When we follow Jesus's example and thank God for the food that we are about to eat and ask that He nourish our bodies in Jesus's name, a transformation takes place, and each person around the table is satisfied and uniquely nourished.

CHAPTER 11

SEED

Throughout both the Old and New Testament, there are numerous references to the word "seed." Contextually, it makes sense because, at the time the Bible was written, it was an agrarian culture.

Farming was a way of life. It was the only way to have food. We have learned in recent chapters God created seed-bearing plants for Adam's consumption. Prior to the Flood, seed-bearing plants were Adam's only food.

God is about life. And He seems to be focused on our consumption of things that produce life. With seed, there is no one- to-one correlation. For example, you do not plant a tomato seed and harvest one tomato. The seed produces multiple times more fruit and provides more harvest than the number of the original seed planted.

In 1 Peter 1:23, He tells us that the Bible is the "incorruptible seed." It is perfect, and it will produce a harvest every time it is planted. When God tells us, "Man does not live by bread alone, but by every word that proceeds out of the mouth of God," there is an important message there.

Years ago, I decided I would plant a garden at my parents' house. I did not want to buy established plants. I chose instead to start the entire garden from seed in my house one hour away. Anticipating planting the garden after the last frost, which typically occurs around April in Virginia, I began planning my garden in January of that year. I bought packets of seeds for the various produce I wanted. I had a few varieties of corn, tomatoes, beans, watermelons, and peppers. My choices were very deliberate.

I purchased sprouting trays and organic soil. My dad built for me an elaborate grow light system out of PVC pipe. My dining room looked like a science lab. I even had a watering schedule. Every day I would check to see if there were any signs of life in the form of a speck of green protruding through the dark, moist dirt. After what seemed like weeks bordering on months, overnight, a brave and resilient sprout poked its head through the soil. I do not know how to describe the feeling. I felt so accomplished and excited. Planting all those seeds, I knew there was a chance some or many would not "take." Before seeing any evidence of success, there were a lot of variables to consider. Was the seed good? Was I watering the dirt enough or too much? Were there enough nutrients in the soil? Were there too many seeds crowded together?

While I didn't have 100% success, I still had success. Appropriately timed, I packed up all the little plants and drove them to my parents' house, where we spent an entire warm, spring Saturday planting them in their designated spots. Now began another waiting season. We waited and watched and tended the tender plants until one day, there appeared a small bloom. It was the most beautiful sign of success. While I was the one who planted the seed, I had no control over the timing of the harvest. As the garden became more established, there were different ways to tend to it. The weeds needed to be pulled. And as the spring and summer became hotter and drier, the garden needed more water. My mom devised a makeshift sprinkler system to combat the long, dry spells. Dad would battle the grass, trying to grow up between the tomato and pepper plants. Often, he would grab the hoe and mound up the dirt around the potatoes. I have lovely memories of being out in the garden with my parents. We were working toward a common goal and chatting. Dad would reminisce about his father, who loved to garden and who, when I was small, had planted a garden in the same patch of land at my parents' house. I'll never forget the advice my grandad gave my mom about planting the potato cuttings. He said you had to wrap them in tissue before you put them in the ground to keep the dirt out of their eyes. Though I was learning to garden as the garden was growing, I knew that I couldn't just put a seed in the ground and forget about it. It needed attention. It needed protection. I planted the seed, but my job wasn't finished until the plant produced the desired fruit.

In Genesis 8:22, the Bible tells us, "As long as the earth endures, seedtime and harvest, cold and heat, summer and winter, day and night will never cease." While this is another example of His grace, that the earth will continue to produce, it's also a message that we should be planting seeds all the time. A cursory glance of this verse, and with my limited knowledge of gardening or botany, I thought the "cold," "winter," and "night" references meant taking time off. They were times when things are dormant. Nothing happens during those cycles. But, after further review, I don't think that's what this verse means. Certain crops do well in the cold. Here in the south, you want your collards touched by a frost. Doing some research years ago, I read that during the day, when the plant was exposed to light, it was busy absorbing the light energy. During the night, it used the stored energy to grow. There is no insignificant time of day or season of the year when it comes to planting seeds. Times when seeds may appear to be inactive, they are still a living thing waiting for the right environment and the right time to come to life.

I read a disturbing statistic the other day from Nutrisend. It stated, "If you eat broccoli today, it's got 50% fewer nutrients in it than it did fifty years ago because of how we grow the food and the depletion of the soil." You can have good seed, but it won't produce if the soil is not good. It feels overwhelming. How can you control those factors that affect your health? Looking at it in the physical, it seems hopeless. In the spiritual sense, you have a relationship with the God who tells the ground what to do. Just like with the grapes becoming wine, we see that food responds to His voice. Maybe the physical battle seems too big; we can't always control how the food is grown, but once it's on our plate, we can talk to the Lord about it.

While all of this makes sense about the physical seeds we expect will produce our food, for the Christian, it also applies to the spiritual seed of the Word of God. The Bible tells us it is the "incorruptible seed." In Isaiah 55:11, God promises, "It is the same with my Word. I send it out, and it always produces fruit. It will accomplish all I want it to, and it will prosper everywhere I send it." As a rookie gardener, if I had a guarantee that every seed I prepared and planted for my garden would produce a harvest, it would be a game-changer. A guaranteed harvest is what the Bible is telling us will happen when we speak His Word.

God wants us to have good success. The Bible tells us in 2 Corinthians 9:10, "He who supplies seed to the sower and bread for food will also supply and increase your store of seed and will enlarge the harvest of your righteousness." You must do something with the seed. You spiritually plant it by speaking it. God's not going to plant it for you. The more seed you plant in good soil, the more harvest you will have.

When we speak God's Word, we are planting a seed that is guaranteed to produce a harvest. Matthew 4:4 tells us, "Man shall not live by bread alone." This is the physical seed. Then the verse continues, "but by every word that proceeds out of the mouth of God." This word is the spiritual seed. Because man is a body, soul, and spirit, he needs both physical and spiritual food.

I was interested in the Hebrew and Greek use of the word "seed." There are seed references in the Garden of Eden; there are seed references in some of the parables, and regarding the Word of God. There are even seed references to Christians in Abraham's lineage. With such a frequently used word in varying contexts, I was curious as to the deeper philosophical or biblical definition of seed. So, I referenced the Strongest NIV Exhaustive Concordance. Brace yourself. Are you ready? It means "a seed." The terms for seed regarding planting, speaking His Word, and being a Christian, all mean roughly the same thing.

What is a seed? According to the research, the first reference to seed in Genesis is the Hebrew word *zera,* which means "seed." The seed mentioned in the "incorruptible seed" used in 1 Peter 1:23 is the Greek word *spora,* which means "seed." From God's perspective, the seed in the Garden and the "incorruptible seed" of the Word of God are viewed as the same thing. A seed is capable of producing life. It is the embryo of a future harvest. Even though it is small, in the right environment, it has tremendous productive capability.

We are Abraham's seed; we speak the seed of the Word of God, and we eat the physical seed that was explicitly designed to fuel our body. All seed can produce life. Here we see the connection among man's body, spirit, and soul again. Seeds produce a harvest in all three areas of man's being. It's not surprising that the physical seed is our food. We must eat every day. But do we speak the Word every day? When we plant a tomato plant, we expect tomatoes. But what are we planting with our words? Do we plant the seed found in His Word regarding our health? How about our food? Do we even know that those seeds are available? His Word is alive and waiting for us to do something with it. We must put it in the right soil.

In Matthew 13, we read about the Parable of the Sower. A farmer went out to sow seed. Some of his seed fell in areas where there was not much soil, others fell among thorns, while others fell on good soil. Where it fell on good ground, it produced a harvest a hundred, sixty or thirty times what was sown. For a gardener, that's exciting!

Toward the end of the hot southern summers when I was a kid, the two sawhorses with a plywood board stretched over them were spilling over with the harvest of tomatoes. Even though my mom canned them, put them in salads, and gave them away, we had accumulated a pile of fresh tomatoes. At this stage, they took on a different purpose. The longer they sat, the softer and mushier they became, which made them perfect for throwing at my sister. The visual impact of an exploding rotten tomato on the back of my fleeing sibling was pure entertainment. When my brothers, sister, and I were all involved, it was warfare. You never knew from which direction a tomato grenade was coming. Oh, the memories!

What kind of spiritual seeds are you planting? Are you confident in what the Word says? Matthew 13:19 reads, "When anyone hears the message about the kingdom and does not understand it, the evil one comes and snatches away what was sown in their heart." Additionally, in verse 25, a man had sowed good seed in his field, "But while everyone was sleeping, his enemy came and sowed weeds." We saw this with Eve in the Garden.

The enemy doesn't want your seed to take root because

he knows that it will produce a fantastic harvest. He uses doubt such as "Did God really say ...?" He uses worry to choke out the Word. If you're focused on the world and on what's happening around you instead of the powerful, spiritual seed, the harvest will be impacted.

When it comes to our food, our focus must be both physical and spiritual. Our bodies are designed to function best on the seed-bearing food God created for us. We consume the produce of the physical seed. We also speak the spiritual seed. Just as important, or maybe, more importantly, our lives reflect our verbal diet. Are you planting spiritual seeds? Are you planting the wrong seeds? There would be nothing worse than planting corn seeds, and green beans grow instead. You didn't get what you expected. If this happened in your physical garden, you wouldn't blame the dirt or the water. You'd know you planted the wrong seed.

It's not a coincidence that the most significant impact on our health is isolated to one area of the body: the mouth. Remember, the Bible says the power of life and death is in the tongue. What are you eating, and what are you speaking?

According to the Bible, seedtime and harvest will always endure. So what seeds are you planting? There will always be seedtime and harvest. We still need to be seedtime minded. After planting my seeds in my dining room garden, every day I would look to see some signs of life. My dad gave me a cartoon he found in the local newspaper where a woman had planted a seed in a flowerpot. Every day she looked at the dirt. The next frame shows her peering at the soil with a magnifying glass. The last frame shows her husband standing beside her while she looked at the dirt. He lovingly tells her, "Be patient." When we plant a seed, there is much anticipation. We know what to look for and what we are expecting. It should be the same when we plant a spiritual seed. Anticipate it. Expect it. He promises it will not return void.

When you understand something, you own it. You can talk about it. You can even teach it. When there is confusion, there is room for shifting or vacillating. You can easily be swayed, or your mind can easily be changed. For example, Eve didn't know what God told her and Adam regarding what they could eat. She had the basis, but she added to it. If she had known fully and was so convinced of the truth, when the enemy asked, "Did God really say...?" She would have been armed and ready to shut him down. That literally would have made all the difference in the world.

We put a lot of responsibility on our food to make us healthy and help us feel good. And it is not misplaced. When we eat food that God didn't create, over time, we don't feel well. But God is telling us that focusing just on our food is only half of the equation. What we plant spiritually with our words, with His Word, is even more critical. So, ask the Lord to give you a verse that fits your situation. When He does, it is your seed. Plant it. Speak it. Keep looking for the harvest that is coming. Remember, a seed does not only produce a fruit. One seed, one verse, will produce a harvest. It produces abundance; it produces life.

By grace, you are a gardener. Between the front and the back cover of your Bible is a treasure trove of seed. Because you are the righteousness of God in Christ Jesus, you live according to the kingdom of God. It's not just about eating. Plant your seeds for the harvest you want to see. Is it health? Then plant the seed. Is it a changed relationship with food? Then plant your seed. Water it with thanksgiving every day, knowing it is guaranteed to produce a harvest. Just like when my family was overrun with tomatoes, your harvest will be so great it will be a blessing to you and to other people.

CHAPTER 12

COMMUNION

Because Adam and Eve disobeyed God and ate the forbidden fruit, sin entered the world. Every person born since that fateful moment is born with a sinful nature. The Lord warned Adam that if they ate of the tree, they would surely die. The moment they ate, the proverbial clock began ticking. We have become accustomed to the numerous markers or stages leading up to physical death. These can be marked with signs of being tired, sick, feeble, having a general decline in health, wrinkles, forgetfulness, and an inexhaustible list of other ailments. They each represent a slow progression toward the end of life. Every day, we attempt to slow the process by eating better, exercising, taking medication, or a myriad of other options. The other death God was warning Adam of was a spiritual death. Very simply, spiritual death is eternal separation from God in Hell.

Christians believe Jesus's death on the cross paid our sin

debt in full. Growing up in church, I was taught this provided us with eternal life after physical death. I don't recall many discussions about how the cross impacted my daily life. From what I do remember, I was told I needed to do good things for other people; I needed to read my Bible; I needed to not put my sister in a headlock; and I needed to attend church every time the doors were opened. I developed a belief that the cross only impacted the spiritual things in my life. Because it determined where I was going to spend eternity, it kicked in once I died.

In the Garden, when they ate the fruit, physical and spiritual punishments were enacted. I began to think about the relationship between the act of eating a physical piece of fruit from the Tree of the Knowledge of Good and Evil and the resulting spiritual consequences. Could this physical-spiritual relationship still be relevant today? Unequivocally, yes.

The answer to our sin debt is and always will be Jesus's death on the cross. His death provided us with salvation. The Greek word for salvation is *sozo*. It means "to heal, restore, deliver, and make whole." This definition is not limited to the spiritual realm. This definition has a broad application in the physical world as well.

Galatians 1:4 states, "who [Jesus] gave himself for our sins, that he might deliver us from this present evil world, according to the will of God and our Father." So, as Christians, shouldn't our attitude about all things related to "this present evil world" be different than the world's view? Shouldn't our perspective about sickness and disease be different? Shouldn't our perspective about food be different?

Because of the blood of Jesus, shouldn't we have an advantage that the world doesn't have?

For example, because of sin, the ground was cursed. Adam had to work to produce the plants to make bread. Genesis 3:18 tells us God promised Adam that thorns would grow where he was attempting to plant his garden. Years later, on the cross, Jesus would wear a crown of thorns on his brow. Thorns were part of the curse. In John 19:2, we are told, "The soldiers twisted together a crown of thorns and put it on his head." Thorns also represent hardship. The hardship was introduced in conjunction with Adam's ability to produce food. Jesus's death took it away. Arguably, a cursed ground would affect the quality of the food produced in that soil. Man is continually trying new and improved methods to battle the thorns and weeds that strangle the plants. Today, food growers manipulate the ground by adding chemicals and genetically modifying seeds to increase the yield. Consequently, our soil is depleted of its nutrients, altering the nutritional composition and quality of all crops that grow. Because of the cross, and the shedding of Jesus's blood in the Garden of Gethsemane, shouldn't our food supply be made whole? In Deuteronomy 28:4-5, those who are in Christ are promised: "Blessed shall be ... the produce of your ground ... Blessed shall be your basket and kneading bowl." What you plant and the food you make is blessed because you are in Christ.

Adam's relationship with food changed. His eating the forbidden fruit introduced struggle and hardships. Without recognizing what we are entitled to and the application of the cross to our food, we, too, are left struggling and experiencing hardships in connection with our nutrition.

In Matthew 4:4, we are told, "Man shall not live on bread alone, but on every word that comes from the mouth of God." We see the same physical and spiritual connection. Here you have reference to physical bread and the spiritual Word of God. Very clearly, God is telling us that we need both in our daily diet.

We see it again in Proverbs 4:22. The words found within the Bible are "Life to those who find them, and health to all their flesh." The spiritual words provide a benefit to your flesh or physical body. Remember, we are body, soul, and spirit. The three are inextricably connected. If only the body and soul are taken care of, then the entire man can still suffer. In other words, when we are focused on only our body and what we eat without the awareness of the spiritual, it is like a three-legged stool with only two legs remaining. Each leg may be strong and sturdy, but the stool can't stand.

As Christians, can't we, because of the blood of Jesus, spiritually "bless" our food and believe that it will be physically beneficial to our body? In the previous chapter, we discussed how Jesus simply thanked His Father for the food, and there was a physical transformation. It multiplied and met the varied nutritional needs of all those present. When we ask Him to bless our meal, we are inviting Him to enhance what the food on its own will do. When the Holy Spirit leads us regarding what to eat, because He knows what we need, then we are never lacking. Following Jesus's example, the physical-spiritual relationship is established.

Further, there's a spiritual and physical aspect of salvation. As Christians, we have been sufficiently taught about the eternal benefits of believing in Jesus's death, burial, and resurrection. But we don't apply it today to the physical.

People are obsessively focused on food providing health and what to eat or what not to eat based on what doctors or the government tell them. It seems to me we should be taking advantage of all the benefits of the cross, but we aren't.

Jesus referred to Himself as the Bread of Life. Since there are no coincidences in the Bible, this is a point worth mentioning. Jesus is the spiritual bread necessitated by the physical bread Adam would have to work to make. For this reason, we use bread or some form of it during the communion service. As Christians, we can benefit from a spiritual and physical power in communion.

The Lord wants you involved in your food. Feeding yourself and your family is a responsibility or privilege that He doesn't want to be delegated to someone else. We see this in the Garden. God created the Garden, then told Adam to tend it. Adam had the opportunity to interact with and get to know where his food was being produced. God wanted him to take an active role in his relationship with his food. Food was an integral part of Adam's life; it was everywhere whenever he wanted it. It is no different for us. But sadly, the relationship for us has become distant and dysfunctional.

By now, we have established that salvation restored the relationship between God and man. Because of the precious blood of Jesus, we can approach God at any time. We can talk to Him whenever and about whatever we want. Because of the robe of righteousness when God sees us, He sees Jesus's perfection. Therefore, when He sees us, it's as if we never sinned. So why is the benefit of the cross not applied or understood concerning our everyday lives? Or, for our purposes here, in connection with our food?

How did salvation affect our physical lives? Sin made us sick. Salvation makes us whole. With all the manipulation and chemical treatments being done to our food, could we not agree that our food is also sick? It lacks in nutrients, and the seeds are modified. There are new items on the store shelves that didn't even exist years ago that our bodies do not recognize as food. Wouldn't salvation make our food whole?

There is no mention in the Bible of having to worry about what you eat. This is a construct of man. Whether we want to admit it or not, we want rules. There is a false safety in rules or at least a promise of a result. For example, if you follow this diet, you can expect to lose a certain number of pounds. The Israelites wanted the Ten Commandments. Jesus came so that the rules were no longer necessary. Rules are part of the law; Christ is the fulfillment of the law.

With all the confusion and conflicting advice surrounding food, isn't it interesting that we use food, or bread, to remember the cross? Again, here we see a spiritual and physical connection or relationship to food.

In Genesis chapter 14, Abram had returned from battle after successfully rescuing his nephew Lot and all of Lot's possessions. In verse 18, Melchizedek, the king of Salem, brought bread and wine to Abram. Here is the first reference to communion. The Bible describes Melchizedek as the "priest of God Most High." The name Melchizedek means "My king is righteous" or "king of righteousness." Incidentally, Salem is a derivative of the Hebrew word Shalom or peace, one of the gifts addressed in a previous chapter. Some Bible scholars believe that "the bread and wine was just an ordinary meal and was in no way related to the NT [New Testament] ordinance of communion." But there are no coincidences, nor are there extraneous or irrelevant details with God.

Back in the Garden, in Genesis 3:19, the Lord told Adam, because he ate from the forbidden tree, "In the sweat of your face you shall eat bread till you return to the ground." As mentioned before, this is the first instance in which bread is mentioned in the Bible. Think about what bread represents to Adam. Every time he eats it, he is reminded of his sin. He is eating bread because of his own choices. The bread represents the worst decision of his entire life. Imagine the sadness and guilt he must feel.

The next mention of bread in the Bible is eleven chapters later in Genesis 14:18, when Melchizedek, king of Salem, brings bread and wine to Abram after a battle is won. The verse reads that Melchizedek gave Abram the bread and wine and blessed him. This instance is unusual because, before this moment, bread was associated with a curse, Adam's curse.

Just for review, *Shalem* or *shalom* means "perfect peace" or "wholeness." The fact that Melchizedek is from Salem is an important point. According to research, "*Shalom*" is taken from the root word *shalam*, which means, "to be safe in mind, body, or estate." It speaks of completeness, fullness, or a type of wholeness. In Israel today, when you say, "*Shalom*," you are saying, "may you be full of well-being" or "may health and prosperity be upon you." It is essential to recognize that the definition of *shalom* does not only indicate a spiritual benefit; there's a physical benefit as well. Isn't it interesting that the King of "*Shalom*" was giving Abram bread?

While watching Adam and Eve leave the Garden forever, God had already set into motion the answer to correct what Adam's sin caused. Many years later, His Son, Jesus, would die to pay the debt. We take the bread of communion to remember.

From a spiritual perspective, is it any coincidence that we are in a bread-avoidance culture? It is trendy to be carb conscious. When people attempt to eat low or no carbohydrates, the first thing they eliminate from the diet is bread. Doing this is understandable, especially since bread is a staple in the standard American diet. Our meals tend to revolve around some variation of bread. When I was growing up, and even still today, my dad will tease my mom after she has placed dinner on the table. If he notices that there is no bread, he will jokingly say, "I guess that means we're having dessert." Bread is one of the favorite parts of a meal. When you go out to a fancy restaurant, they bring you a basket of bread. This does not typically happen at your local fast-food joint.

Our language even includes creative uses of the word "bread." For example, when you have a meal with someone, you "break bread together." There is a specific connotation to that phrase. Asking someone if they would like to "break a carrot stick together" doesn't have the same effect, and you'd probably receive a very quick and polite "No, thank you."

The "greatest thing since sliced bread" idiom is used to describe something that is so much better or easier. We can all agree that, compared to the old flash-bulb cameras and several other devices, our cell phone is the "greatest thing since sliced bread."

When we talk about money or our economic productivity, we often will use the words "bread" or "dough." According to Rabbi Daniel Lapin, "In the tabernacle or the temple, there is a special place on which loaves of bread are placed to signify the kickstart of Israel's economy."

In Matthew 6:11, Jesus instructs us how to pray and includes a verbatim request for bread. In the Lord's Prayer, we recite, "Give us this day our daily bread." This bread is our daily answer.

Bread is a staple in our culture. It is on our plates, and it's in our language. Even with the above examples, we tend to focus on bread in the physical sense. Yet, in the spiritual sense, we have a greater need for it.

In Matthew 4:3, Jesus was led into the wilderness by the Spirit to be tempted by the devil. Now, this is the same devil that approached the woman in the Garden. After fasting 40 days and nights, Jesus was hungry. When Jesus was at his weakest due to hunger, the devil approached Him, saying, "If You are the Son of God, command that these stones become bread." Jesus replied, "It is written that man shall not live by bread alone, but by every word that proceeds from the mouth of the God." Notice how Satan was trying to shift Jesus's focus to only the physical benefit of bread. Eating bread would temporarily remove His hunger. Jesus's response to include both the physical and the spiritual perspectives defeated the enemy.

This response is also the same language God told the Israelites in Deuteronomy 8:3. "So He humbled you, allowed you to hunger, and fed you with manna which you did not know nor did your fathers know, that He might make you know that man shall not live by bread alone; but man lives by every word that proceeds from the mouth of the Lord." Our success with anything, including our health and nutrition, must include both the physical and spiritual focus.

Jesus's temptation is an interesting moment. Stones represent man's effort. For example, the Ten Commandments were written on two stone tablets. Many people believe they must work for their salvation instead of relying on the work of the cross. Self-effort cannot, nor will it ever bring shalom. But the bread will. Satan was tempting Jesus to convert stones into bread. From the symbolic standpoint, stones could never be the basis of the bread. Man's effort could never serve as a sufficient starting point. If Jesus converted stones into bread, then shalom would always be based on the foundation of self-effort. Our salvation is in no way attributed to or based on stone. Our salvation or shalom is solely and completely based on the sacrifice of Jesus on the cross. His finished work is complete, and because of that, we are also complete. Nothing we do can add to or take away from our salvation.

In 1 Corinthians 11:24 and 26, Jesus handed the disciples the bread and said, "Take, eat; this is My body broken for you; do this in remembrance of Me. ... For as often as you eat this bread and drink this cup, you shall proclaim the Lord's death until He comes." This is why bread is part of the communion ceremony. Not just out of ritual, but to receive all the benefits of the cross.

I heard a story of a woman who got up one Sunday morning and got dressed, drove herself to church, and entered the sanctuary. She noticed the accouterments of the communion ceremony were positioned at the front of the church. The woman immediately turned around, exited the church, and drove home. When asked about why she left, she explained that it was just communion and not a church service. This missed opportunity happens frequently.

When you consume the bread during communion, you are consuming all the physical and spiritual benefits and blessings Jesus died on the cross for you to have. The bread represents everything His physical body endured. It was whipped so that you can be healed. His body took on every sickness and every disease so that you do not have to. From a nutritional standpoint, the health status of our body typically drives many of our food decisions and choices. We alter our diet to avoid sickness and to recover when we are sick. We equate our health with food. And it is true. But for most Christians, we forgo the spiritual benefit of the cross, which will provide an even more significant benefit to our body physically.

In communion, bread represents the blessing. We do not live under the curse anymore. We can live free. But just because we can live this way does not mean that many Christians do. I heard the story of a man who had a million dollars in the bank. He lived in abject poverty. He barely had enough to eat, and his home was in shambles. All the while, he had the money in the bank though he did not know it was there. It was left in an account set up in his name after the death of a distant relative whom he never knew. If he knew there was money that belonged to him, it would change the way he lived. It would change the decisions he made. He was a millionaire all this time, yet he lived in poverty. He made poverty decisions because it is who he thought he was. He did not know the truth. Sadly, he didn't benefit from who he was. He was a millionaire with a poverty mindset making poverty decisions.

It is the same with us as Christians. The Bible is our money in the bank. There are advantages we have because of the finished work of the cross. Yet many Christians live as if they are still struggling under the sin debt. They believe they are cursed. They know they are saved; they are just trying to hang on until Jesus comes back. They think once they get to heaven, everything will be better, "in the sweet by and by." But as we have seen with Melchizedek, the blessings he provided to Abram were physical and available to Abram at that very moment.

The bread Adam was told he would have to make after the Garden represents work. Compared to the ease of picking fruit from the trees he didn't plant, having to make your bread required a lot of work. Think about it. You had to grow the grain. You had to harvest and thresh the grain. Then you had to work it with your hands and mix it with water to make it into bread. Eating would require time and patience. Picking a kumquat was so much easier.

When it comes to food today, many of us still live like Adam. We put a lot of thought, worry, and effort into what we eat. Yet, the Lord has taken that away from us. Bread is the food of God. He told Adam to make it. He tells us to eat it to remember the cross and live in the blessings.

We see Adam's mindset with the Israelites. In Deuteronomy 8:9-10, the Lord describes the Promised Land as a "land in which you will eat bread without scarcity, in which you will lack nothing. ... When you have eaten and are full, then you shall bless the Lord your God for the good land He has given you." God took the Israelites out of Egypt, a place where they were slaves. In Numbers 11:4-5, while wandering in the Wilderness, the Israelites complained to Moses about the manna God was providing. We read, "Meanwhile, the rabble among them had a strong craving for other food, and again the Israelites wept and said, 'Who will feed us meat? We remember the fish we ate freely in Egypt, along with the cucumbers, melons, leeks, onions, and garlic.'" Notice their desire to be able to "eat freely." They didn't care that the menu they were fondly remembering came with extremely harsh physical labor. In Egypt, they had to work for their food. Their mentality was of a laborer. It was connected to their self- effort. God was taking them to the Promised Land flowing with milk and honey, where they would have vineyards they didn't plant.

In Exodus 16:3, the Israelites complained: "If only we had died by the Lord's hand in the land of Egypt!" they said.

"There we sat by pots of meat and ate our fill of bread, but you have brought us into this desert to starve this whole assembly to death!" The provision of bread came with a price, just like with Adam. They had to work for it. Jesus is making the distinction that He has bread that provides life, and it requires no effort on our part. Just like with the Israelites living in Egypt, the Lord has a Promised Land waiting for you.

The Bread of Life is the gift. Jesus declares in John 6:48-51, "I am the Bread of Life. Your fathers ate the manna in the wilderness and are dead. This is the bread which comes down from heaven, that one may eat of it and not die. I am the living bread which came down from heaven. If anyone eats of this bread, he will live forever; and the bread that I shall give is My flesh, which I shall give for the life of the world." In verse 53, He tells us that taking communion is part of the relationship with Him. He says, "Most assuredly, I say to you, unless you eat the flesh of the Son of Man and drink His blood, you have no life in you. Whoever eats My flesh and drinks My blood has eternal life, and I will raise him up at the last day. For My flesh is food indeed, and My blood is drink indeed. He who eats My flesh and drinks My blood abides in Me, and I in him."

There is a physical and spiritual aspect of bread; however, nutritionists, scientists, and the like focus only on the physical side of the coin. But to the Christian, bread has a vital spiritual element that is most often overlooked or never realized. Even if you eliminated it from your diet, you still need the spiritual. The spiritual benefits cannot be achieved by anything else. There's no substitute for Jesus, the Bread of Life.

The Lord told Adam not to eat the fruit, or he would die. Now He is telling us that by eating the Bread, we will live. There's no work associated with Jesus's form of bread. The Lord told Adam, "don't eat," but he did it anyway. Now, to live in the blessings of the cross resulting from the payment of the sin debt in full, He tells us, "just eat" and eat "often." In 1 Corinthians 11:26, we read, "For as often as you eat this bread and drink the cup, you proclaim the Lord's death until he comes."

Because of what happened to Eve in the Garden, there is an aspect of bread that needs to be discussed. In Leviticus 2:11, the Scriptures tell us, "No grain offering which you bring to the Lord shall be made with leaven, for you shall burn no leaven nor any honey in any offering to the Lord made by fire."

In Matthew 16:6, Jesus cautioned His disciples, "Take heed and beware of the leaven of the Pharisees and the Sadducees." Growing up, I heard a lot of preaching about the Pharisees. They were dogmatic about their adherence to the law. It was legalism at its most extreme. I can remember sitting in a Sunday School class. The teacher was trying to explain to a group of uninterested nine and ten-year-olds who the Pharisees and Sadducees were. The teacher taught that both groups were against Jesus. Neither liked the way He did things.

The Pharisees were upset because Jesus broke their laws by healing people and getting an ox out of a ditch, none of which you could do on the Sabbath. I remember the teacher saying the Sadducees were "sad-u- see." I know. A bit corny, but I never forgot it. I just thought they were people in town who always appeared sad. It wasn't until recently that I understood they were the group during Jesus' time on earth who followed a doctrine of humanism. They discounted Jesus's supernatural miracles and His teachings, believing that everything could be explained by using science. And that got me thinking. The science of nutrition states the same thing.

Isn't this the crux of the problem with nutrition and food choices today? If you can't prove it by scientific means, then it either doesn't exist or is not valid. Here is the same conflict. The Bible says something about food and nutrition, but Christians tend to believe what science is saying more. Don't we want the supernatural in our nutrition? How can science prove what God says faith can do? This way of thinking discounts the spiritual aspect of food.

God's Word refers to the erroneous teachings of Pharisees and Sadducees as "leaven." So, if Jesus is our "grain offering," then He alone is enough. When we add erroneous teachings to what Jesus did on the cross, we are adding leaven to the grain. His finished work is enough and is why unleavened bread is used for communion. It is a stand-alone work. The Lord did not need us to add to the finished work. If that were the case, then the cross would be unfinished. It would be for nothing really if we still need to work to make it better or more effective. Incidentally, as we have discussed earlier, Eve added to God's instructions. She added to His Word and made it more complicated than it needed to be. This addition was a contributing factor to her confusion and her vulnerability to the serpent. The serpent didn't lie. He didn't give her nutritional facts and figures. He simply nudged her in the direction she was already headed by asking, "Did God really say ...?"

The wafer cracker used during the communion service is typically unleavened bread. Often, you will see the Hebrew matzah cracker used and is for a significant reason. There is no yeast, or leaven, in the cracker. Also, the appearance of the cracker is significant. If you look at the matzah cracker, there are little burnt or brown linear markings all over it. These marks represent two important points. First, Jesus was the perfect sacrifice that was exposed to the fiery wrath of His Father when He took on all our sin. Second, the lines on the matzah also represent the stripes on Jesus's body because of the scourging at the whipping post. These two points reinforce the meaning when you read, "By His stripes, you are healed."

When you realize Christ redeemed you from every curse, that means every curse that was proclaimed in the Garden, which includes the cursed ground and having to work for your food. We also became the craving of the enemy. We are warned of this in 1 Peter 5:8, which tells us to "Be alert and of sober mind. Your enemy the devil prowls around like a roaring lion looking for someone to devour."

Curses shouldn't apply to Christians anymore since the cross paid for everything. God wants us to enjoy every blessing that was paid for at the cross. So, it would behoove us to become familiar with all the blessings to which we are entitled. Living in ignorance is no different than the poverty-stricken millionaire we read about earlier. He was living far beneath his potential. Sadly, so are we.

It has been shown that relying on science can lead to misinformation. If you read scientific studies, you find there typically is a bias in the reporting of the data to the benefit of the person or organization funding the study. From those scientific findings in connection with food, nutrition guidelines and proclamations are developed. This bias can be just like blending Jesus and leaven.

What does the Bible say about food? Isn't that all we need to know? The struggle to navigate through the ever-changing information of what to eat and what not to eat is overwhelming. It is understandable that when it comes to food, most people are sad-you-see? See what I did there?

Why is Jesus represented as bread? In the Garden, God told Adam he would now have to toil for his food. Bread would be the result of Adam's struggle and work. But when we take communion, when we eat the bread, we are acknowledging that Jesus is the replacement. Because the curse has been removed from our lives, we don't have to rely on work. The bread in communion also represents the new bread. We don't receive righteousness through works, which Adam's bread represents. We receive it by faith in Jesus, which the communion bread represents. In Romans 3:23-25, we read, "For all have sinned and fall short of the glory of God, and all are justified freely by his grace through the redemption that came by Christ Jesus. God presented Christ as a sacrifice of atonement, through the shedding of his blood — to be received by faith."

Additionally, in Ephesians 2:8-9, the Bible reads, "For by grace you have been saved through faith. And this is not your own doing; it is the gift of God, not a result of works, so that no one may boast." So, when we partake of communion, we are acknowledging the sacrifice of Jesus. In Isaiah 53:5, we read that "But he was wounded for our transgressions, he was bruised for our iniquities ... and with his stripes we are healed."

There is power in the bread of communion. Not because of the physical makeup of the bread, but the spiritual aspect that the communion wafer represents. The Bread of Life brings health, healing, and all the other aspects of salvation, which were not necessary until Adam and Eve sinned.

When Jesus fed the 5,000 people, there were twelve baskets of bread left over. While offering different perspectives and details on this story, each of the gospel authors included the twelve leftover baskets into their account. Research tells us twelve is a perfect number that represents "material and spiritual food." What the 5,000 consumed that day provided both physical and spiritual nutrition.

In Matthew 14:20, we read that there were twelve baskets of broken pieces. Since no detail is irrelevant in God's Word, compare this to Matthew 26:26 regarding the Last Supper. Jesus took the bread, gave thanks, broke it, and gave it to his disciples.

When someone tells the story commonly referred to as "The Feeding of the 5,000," they always speak of how a little boy gave his lunch of five loaves and two fish to feed the crowd. But the mention of the boy is only in John's account. I believe this is a point worth making. When it comes to food, the source of the food is not as important. What is essential and deemed worth mentioning by all four gospel authors is that the food was in Jesus's hands, and He gave thanks to His Father. No matter the account, the starting point of the miracle is Jesus. That's when the food changed.

The same is true for us when we take communion. All that matters is Jesus. When we partake of the bread during the ceremony, just as in feeding the 5,000 people, with Jesus, everything changes. Our nutritional and health needs are met. Communion is incredibly powerful. The enemy knows of the power. Otherwise, he would not be so determined to convince Christians and church leaders, for that matter, that it's irrelevant today. Do as Jesus instructed His disciples: Eat the bread often.

AFTERWORD

This book has been the culmination of a search for answers to food and nutrition questions I have held for several years. Though I have a substantial library related to food and health, I have found myself frustrated, overwhelmed, and discouraged with finding the right approach to feed my body. What I eat is genuinely my responsibility. Yet, there is so much riding on getting the diet and nutrition right. If you don't eat correctly, you are more likely to develop a disease. You are more likely to feel bad, get sick, gain weight, or even die. Those are steep consequences that most people do not want to experience. So why does the information seem to be so confusing and so wrong? It is frequently changing. The entire process feels like an exercise of trial and error with costly consequences. The best we can do is hope to have less trial and little to no error. But who knows how to do that?

Through the years, I began to wonder, if God created food for Adam, then what was and is God's perspective about food? If He made food for His only companion, then He should have something to say about it. If He is the same yesterday, today and forever, then His perspective shouldn't change. So how God felt about food on that day of Creation or in the Garden should still be how He feels today, right? What I realized is God's perspective about food is less about food and more about His precious Son, Jesus. When Adam was in the Garden, food was a big part of the welcome kit. When Adam sinned, the relationship to God and to food changed. So, if the relationship to God is reconciled, then shouldn't the relationship to food be reconciled as well? What if the two are not mutually exclusive?

When God was telling Adam what his punishment would be, He immediately enacted a plan to reconnect with man; to re-establish the cherished relationship. Because Adam ate the forbidden fruit, which ushered in the physical and spiritual consequences of sin, God immediately introduced the solution: His Son, Jesus. Though Adam wasn't aware of any of this, God told Adam he would now have to make bread. Adam's bread represented his sin consequences. Jesus, the Bread of Life, would be Adam's answer.

Inadvertently, Adam was developing a new relationship, and that was with food. It became a primary focus for survival and fuel. There was a dependency on the bread. Similarly, for the Christian, we are invited to depend on the Bread of Life for everything we need for our survival. Yet, we still need to eat every day.

For this new relationship with food to be possible, God gave us eight additional gifts that would change our relationship with Him and, arguably, as a byproduct, with our food. He gave us grace that we would receive his kindness and all the benefits of the relationship with Him. He gave us righteousness so we can come boldly to the throne of grace, where all our answers are waiting. When we rest in the finished work of the cross, we are functioning in grace. We are no longer separated from Him because we wear the robe of righteousness. When He sees us, He only sees His sinless Son, Jesus. God gave us His wisdom to always know what to do when we don't know what to do. His wisdom allows us to navigate this world and make food and dietary decisions that are best for us, irrespective of what other authorities say. He gives us the power to use our words and to plant spiritual seeds for a harvest of health. He gives us peace or shalom, which is salvation. Peace is all-inclusive. It covers everything from health to rest. With peace, we have wholeness. Finally, He gives us the powerful and life-changing privilege of communion. Communion is a precious reminder of all Jesus did on the cross. There is healing power in communion. While food plays a part in our health, it is secondary to the relationship with Jesus. We typically look to food to do all the things that Jesus has already done for us on the cross.

This book is not about rules regarding how to eat or what to eat. Instead, it is intended to be a thought-provoking look into what the Bible has to say about food. Considering the Bible is a manual for successful living, I believe the topic should be researched. I hope the information on these pages challenge your current way of thinking about food and encourage you to begin to recognize both the physical and spiritual benefits food provides. Our culture is continually preaching to us about the physical benefits. But in kingdom living, the spiritual is so much more powerful. It's the spiritual side of the coin we have been missing. Jesus's death doesn't only determine where we will spend eternity when we die. It influences and changes factors of how we live daily. One of those daily considerations is food. We are becoming more and more knowledgeable about food and what it does for the body, but as a culture, we are becoming sicker and sicker. Health care costs are soaring. People are struggling financially because of health issues. Some crucial part of the solution must be missing. I believe it is our awareness of who we are in Christ and how that changes the relationship to food.

Food was originally intended to be good and pleasing to the sight. We look at food today as fuel. But God didn't explicitly assign food the responsibility of healing our bodies. In all the healings He performed, not once did He prescribe kale or any other food for that matter. Instead, He went to the cross and took away every sickness and disease. He gave us His Word that we can speak, which "provides life to all who find it and health to all their flesh." No matter what the tv commercials, nutritionists, doctors, and government tell you, food can't do all of that. What food item can provide health to all your flesh? Hebrews 4:12 tells us, "... the word of God is alive and active. Sharper than any double- edged sword, it penetrates even to dividing soul and spirit, joints and marrow ..." The Word of God has an impact on our physical bodies.

There's no doubt that the original relationship God had with Adam involved food. Food was everywhere. Adam probably ate it while he and God were talking. Even if he wasn't eating, food surrounded them when they walked in the Garden together. Because of the cross, we can return to that relationship. Food can be there. It can be a part of our life, but not our entire focus. Each time we eat, let it serve as an invitation to talk to your Great Physician, your El Shaddai, your Nourisher. Invite Him into your food choices. He knows you are trying to decipher conflicting messages from the food industry and from those who are out to make a profit. He knows you are concerned about health issues that run in your family or you are currently experiencing today. We have the wisdom to know what to do. And the beauty is that your wisdom will be and look differently than anyone else's wisdom because He knows you individually and personally. We all have different needs He has promised to meet. Because He is the Great Shepherd, we do not lack. We don't have deficiencies. Our needs are met, and that includes nutritional needs as well.

One of the challenges for me in writing this book was deciding whether I was going to take Him at His Word. Contrary to my training, was I going to believe what the Bible said about how to eat? Additionally, was I going to incorporate my research into my daily life? What I found was a respite from struggle when I let Him reignite a new perspective for His original gift. He wants you to step into a deeper relationship with Him and trust Him to develop your new and healthy relationship with food. This book is an invitation for you also to take a stand. Are you going to take your heavenly Father at His Word, or are you going to continue to be tossed about? All the responsibilities and expectations we have assigned to food belong to Jesus. He's already done His part.

When we say a blessing over the food right before we eat, don't let it be a quick, thoughtless recitation. You, the blessing giver, are speaking life into the food. You are changing what that meal is going to do for you, and all those gathered around your table. It is a responsibility and privilege to bless the food. When Jesus gave thanks spiritual and physical food miracles happened. He tells us we have that same power when we use His name.

Know that, because of the cross, you have inherited grace, righteousness, faith, peace, wisdom, thanksgiving, seeds, and the right to partake in communion. None of this is yours because of what you did or who you are. It is because of Jesus's willingness to give His life for you. Your health matters to your Creator, and you have a calling on your life. You wouldn't be reading this book otherwise. To fully realize your calling, you must have fuel; you must be healthy. That was the purpose of the food God created. But even more, is the relationship with Jesus and the finished work of the cross that entitles you to a radically new way of thinking. Let Jesus be your medicine. He'll guide you regarding your food. He'll equip you to do what you need to do if changes need to be made. You rest in Him and let Him care for you. He has already told us man doesn't live by bread alone. He lives by every word that proceeds out of the mouth of God. It seems to me we should know what God says about food. Once we know this, we should start feeding on it. Then we can do what God told Adam to do in the Garden, "Eat freely."

FOOTNOTES

CHAPTER 3

1. Julie Beck, "More Than Half of What Americans Eat Is 'Ultra-Processed,'" The Atlantic, March 10, 2016, https://www.theatlantic.com/health/archive/2016/03/more-than-half-ofwhat-americans-eat-is-ultra-processed/472791/.

CHAPTER 4

1. Kate Bratskeir, "Kraft American Cheese Singles Have Been Labeled a Health Food by Professional Nutritionists (Not as a Joke)," Huffington Post, March 18, 2015, https://www.huffpost.com/entry/kraft-singles-kids-eat-right_n_6879658.

CHAPTER 7

1. Kris Gunners, "Top 10 Benefits of Eating Eggs", Healthline, June 28, 2018, https://www.healthline.com/nutrition/10-proven-health-benefits-of-eggs#section5

CHAPTER 9

1. "The Secrets Behind Your Grocery Store's Layout," Real Simple, February 14, 2018, https://www.realsimple.com/food-recipes/shopping-storing/more-shopping-storing/ grocery-store-layout
2. Peter Economy, "10 Top New Year's Resolutions for Success and Happiness in 2020," Inc.com, December 30, 2019, https://www.inc.com/peter-economy/10-top-new- years-resolutions-for-success-happiness-in-2020.html

CHAPTER 10

1. Gretchen Livingston, "Family Size Among Mothers," Pew Research Center, May 7, 2015, https://www.pewsocialtrends.org/2015/05/07/family-size-among-mothers/

ABOUT THE AUTHOR

Karen Brooks can usually be found researching and writing about food and the human body. She graduated from the College of William and Mary in Virginia and Summa Cum Laude with a Master's degree in Nutrition and Human Performance from Logan University. Karen is an avid reader, fitness enthusiast and trial and error cook. She splits her time between NC and VA with her husband, Chris.

karenbrookslife.com

Made in the USA
Monee, IL
14 February 2021

60419084R00132